Organ Transplants

Making the Most of Your Gift of Life

DISCARD

Organ Transplants

Making the Most of Your Gift of Life

Robert Finn

O'REILLY®

Beijing • Cambridge • Farnham • Köln • Paris • Sebastopol • Taipei • Tokyo

Organ Transplants: Making the Most of Your Gift of Life
by Robert Finn

Copyright © 2000 Robert Finn. All rights reserved.
Printed in the United States of America.

Published by O'Reilly & Associates, Inc., 101 Morris Street, Sebastopol, CA 95472.

Editor: Linda Lamb

Production Editor: Sarah Jane Shangraw

Cover Design: Kathleen Wilson, Ellie Volckhausen, and Edie Freedman

Printing History:

      January 2000: First Edition

Library of Congress CIP data is available at: *http://www.oreilly.com/catalog/organtran*

ISBN: 1-56592-634-X

[M]

Dedicated to organ donors everywhere.

Table of Contents

Foreword

LOOKING AT THOSE LONG, AND LENGTHENING, waiting lists for organs and tissues is, I imagine, one of the most agonizing experiences a sick person can have.

Knowing that at the end of it a new life is waiting and yet having to get through every day until then, never knowing when that moment will come, could undermine anyone's morale.

Let's remember, however, those lists are growing not because there are fewer donors but because new, and still developing, techniques can cure people who even a few years ago had no chance. People who were considered far too old, too young, or too sick for a transplant are now regularly being given a second chance at life.

Those transplants are working better too. These are not experimental procedures any more. Tens of thousands of people all over the world are living healthy, productive lives with new hearts or corneas or lungs. Unlike other serious illnesses, where rehabilitation is typically painfully slow, these patients surprisingly often bounce back to life, with a sparkle in their eyes that shows they feel they have been reborn.

Time and again when talking to recipients, I hear someone who has been living like an invalid say, "I've never felt better in my life."

Better still, unlike almost every other major public issue, there is no significant body of opinion opposing transplants. Every survey shows the overwhelming majority of Americans are in favor. Most say they would donate a loved one's organs and tissue.

The tragic part is that, when the time for a decision about donation comes, only a minority of people who support transplants in theory can bring themselves to do it in practice. This is not hypocrisy. They arrive at the hospital to find someone they love is dead or dying, and to be asked at this shattering time to make a decision in favor of something they have never seriously thought of before is just too much. Emotionally overwhelmed, often unable to talk it over in time with other members of the family, grappling with the mystery of death, many people just can't say yes.

But this too is hopeful. If the reason for refusing to donate is due not to any deep-seated opposition but rather to lack of preparation, the solution is equally clear: we must do everything we can to make sure, long before any tragedy occurs, that people are aware of the life-giving power they have in their hands. The average decision to donate produces three or four organs. That means the families of potential donors can save three or four other families from the devastation they themselves are going through or, in effect, they can condemn them to a lifetime of sorrow. Once they have realized clearly that is the choice they face, it's difficult to imagine most people would do otherwise.

Thousands of people in healthcare are working day in and day out to make this choice clear, through advertising, talks, newspaper articles, community services, notices on the Web, videos—in short, by using every avenue the communications age has opened up.

No doubt we all need to do more, and use more imagination in what we do, to translate good intentions into good behavior. But time is working for us. More and more people now see organ and tissue transplants not as something horrifying, disrespectful, or something they'd prefer to leave to others, but quite simply as the natural thing to do.

Robert Finn's book, grounded as it is on the thoughts and behavior of people of all kinds who find themselves confronting the extraordinary achievements of modern medicine, is another valuable stepping stone on the way to that goal.

—Reg Green
Author of *The Nicholas Effect: A Boy's Gift to the World*
Founder, The Nicholas Green Foundation

Preface

THIS BOOK IS INTENDED FOR ANYONE who may need an organ or tissue transplant, or anyone helping such a person make medical decisions. Sometimes the person who is ill is too wrapped up in pain, worry, and fear to be able to focus clearly on his or her medical options. Sometimes the illness is so severe that it renders the patient unable to make critical medical decisions. It falls then to a family member or trusted friend, working in cooperation with medical professionals, to identify the decisions to be made and to present them clearly to the patient (when possible) or to actually make those decisions (when necessary and with the patient's assent).

The world of transplantation may seem strange and foreign to someone entering it for the first time. People who live in that world seem to speak a language all their own, and they have some awfully strange customs and concerns as well. This book will serve as a guide book to that world. You'll learn what to expect during your journey through transplantation, and you'll learn what to do if you encounter problems.

While this book contains a great deal of medical information, it is meant merely to supplement and not to substitute for advice from medical professionals. Medical science evolves and advances constantly, and some medical details go out of date rapidly. In addition, different organ transplant programs have different ways of doing things. On top of that, I am a journalist and not a physician. Although the publishers and I have diligently endeavored to ensure that all material was accurate at the time it was published, errors may remain, and you should consult medical professionals before adopting procedures or treatments discussed in this book. Use this book as a framework on which to build your knowledge about organ transplantation, and add to that framework with up-to-date information from other sources, including your own research and members of your transplant team.

About the people in this book

In researching this book, I interviewed dozens of people intimately involved in the world of transplantation, including donors, recipients, physicians, nurses, social workers, and other transplant professionals. Their words read like dispatches from the foot soldiers of a medical revolution.

You will find much of what they say to be fascinating and relevant, but you'll also find differing experiences and differing opinions. Human beings are complex biological organisms, but more than that, we all have a deeply spiritual dimension as well. People who receive transplants have different backgrounds, different personalities, and different medical conditions. Medical professionals often disagree on diagnosis and treatment. For those reasons, every person's experience with transplant is unique, and I urge you to keep that in mind as you read their personal accounts. As the saying goes, "Your mileage may vary."

There are no fictional or composite characters in this book. Although the people quoted here were offered anonymity through the use of pseudonyms, every one of them chose to use his or her real name.

Organization of this book

This book is organized so that you may either read it straight through or go directly to the chapter that contains subjects of interest. If you are not already familiar with the world of transplantation, however, it's probably a good idea to start off by reading Chapters 1, 2, and 3.

Chapter 1, *Considering a Transplant*, describes how to make decisions about transplant and presents some critical data. The chapter also contains sections on what many religions think about organ transplant and donation, and demolishes a number of pernicious myths.

Chapter 2, *The System*, describes how individual hospitals, local and regional organ procurement organizations, and the United Network for Organ Sharing (the most important national transplant organization in the US) work together. Here you'll also find general information on how transplant teams evaluate potential candidates for transplant.

Chapter 3, *The Wait*, describes how donor organs are matched with recipients, how the immune system can cause rejection, and how people awaiting transplant can approach this most difficult time.

Chapter 4, *Heart and Lung Transplants*, discusses what sort of people are considered for heart, lung, or heart-lung transplants, and it describes what happens before, during, and after surgery.

Chapter 5, *Liver Transplants*, discusses what sort of people are considered for liver transplants, and it describes what happens before, during, and after surgery.

Chapter 6, *Kidney and Pancreas Transplants*, discusses what sort of people are considered for kidney, pancreas, or kidney-pancreas transplants, and it describes what happens before, during, and after surgery.

Chapter 7, *Other Transplants*, discusses transplants of the bone marrow, corneas, intestines, limbs, skin, and other organs and tissues.

Chapter 8, *Anti-Rejection Drugs*, discusses what rejection is and how it is controlled and treated. It goes into a bit of detail on each of the standard immunosuppressive drugs, describing what they do and what side effects they may have.

Chapter 9, *Living with a Transplant*, discusses how to manage your health after transplant. There's information on keeping your medications straight, making sure you get proper treatment in an emergency room, how to keep from getting infections, and how to live life with gusto as a transplant recipient. There's also some information on cancer, since people taking immunosuppressive medication are at higher risk for some forms of this disease.

Chapter 10, *Emotional Responses*, discusses the range of emotions that transplant recipients and their families experience while riding the transplant roller coaster, and how to deal with them.

Chapter 11, *Family and Support*, discusses how the transplant experience affects couples, children, and whole families, and provides pointers to some of the many avenues for emotional support.

Chapter 12, *Transplants in Children*, discusses some of the special considerations for pediatric transplant recipients.

Chapter 13, *Living Donors*, discusses the advantages and disadvantages for both donors and recipients of living-donor organ transplants.

Chapter 14, *Donors and Recipients*, discusses the remarkable connection between organ donors, their families, and transplant recipients. It examines the difficult and controversial issue of whether donors and recipients should attempt to contact each other. And it describes the opportunities for involvement if you wish to participate in efforts to increase organ donation rates.

Chapter 15, *Financial Issues*, discusses options for funding transplant surgery, which is often extremely expensive. A lifetime of immunosuppressive medication is also quite costly, but there are some ways those costs can be reduced.

Chapter 16, *Traveling for Treatment*, discusses strategies for getting to the hospital that will be performing your transplant. This can be especially challenging if you don't live near a big city with a major medical center.

Chapter 17, *The Future of Transplantation*, discusses how the field may change in the next ten to twenty years. Scientists and physicians are engaged in a great deal of innovative research, some quite controversial, that may make transplantation an option for many more people, and may even make it unnecessary for some.

The appendix, *Resources*, collects in a single location an annotated list of resources related to organ transplants.

Acknowledgments

This book owes a great deal to a great many people. Once again I am pleased to reserve my highest praise for Linda Lamb, editor of the Patient-Centered Guides series. Her good nature helped make this project a delight from beginning to end, and her perceptive editorial comments are reflected on every page.

I'd also like to thank everyone else at O'Reilly & Associates, especially Carol Wenmoth, Shawnde Paull, Lisa Olson, and Leili Eghbal, who worked so hard to get this book to its readers, and Katherine Wilkinson, who did such a wonderful job on the index.

Justin Finn provided valuable research services. And I can't possibly say enough about Linda Goetz and her crew at Coast Lines Secretarial—Sylvia Allen and Noreen Ferrera—who patiently transcribed many hours of interviews.

One of the amazing delights of science and medical journalism is that so many busy people prove willing to spend so much time telling their stories. I thank everyone who generously shared their expertise, who revealed intimate details of their medical histories, who reviewed early versions of manuscript and uncovered many errors, and who provided various other forms of assistance, large and small. In particular, I'd like to thank JoLayna Arndt; Rae Ann Hopkins Berry, LCSW; John and Suzan Best; Mary Waldmann Boucher, RN; Michael, Julie, and Morgan Browning; Mary E. Burge, LCSW; Alice Chang, MSW; Kathy L. Coffman, MD; Donald C. Dafoe, MD; Kathryn M. Flynn; Jim Gleason; Larry S. Goldman, MD; Reg Green; Steve Hon; Melanie Horne; Sharon A. Hunt, MD; Emmet B. Keeffe, MD, Lisa G. Levin, RN, MS; Kathleen Martin, MSW; Deborah Anne Mast; Stacey McCandlish, MSW; Gary McMahan; Joan Miller, RN; Randall E. Morris, MD; Lori Noyes, RN, BSN; Jeffrey D. Punch, MD; Steven W. Rahn; Ivan R. Schwab, MD; Fred Sohl; Ruth SoRelle; Dave and Linda Souza; James Theodore, MD; Randall Vagelos, MD; Michael Wachs, MD; Kristin Weidenbach; and Donna Henry Wright, JD.

I also must thank the many people who participate in the valuable TRNS-PLT mailing list. I have learned an enormous amount by lurking in that forum.

Despite the contributions of so many people to this book, it's likely that some errors remain. Those errors are my own.

Finally, I'd like to thank Joanne Cosmos Finn, my dear wife. Her love and support are a constant source of comfort and inspiration, and this book simply could not have been written without her.

CHAPTER 1

Considering a Transplant

CHANCES ARE, YOU'RE READING THIS BOOK because you or a loved one has recently been handed some devastating news. In all likelihood, you've been suffering serious illness for some time, and your doctor may have recently informed you that there's little more she can do short of surgery to treat your heart, lung, kidney, or liver disease. Now your only possibility of living a normal life is a transplant.

If you're in your 40s or older, you probably remember when organ transplants were front-page news, when both the doctors who performed transplants and the patients who received organs became household names around the world. The good news about organ transplantation is that almost all organ and tissue transplants are now fairly routine. Some major medical centers perform more kidney transplants than appendectomies. Heart transplants are no longer especially challenging to surgeons, and even liver transplants are no longer exotic or experimental and can be done at more than 100 medical centers nationwide.

The even better news about organ transplants is that they do work miracles. People who have been in ill health for years often describe a feeling of being reborn after a transplant. After suffering a debilitating illness that often results in a highly circumscribed existence under the ever present shadow of imminent death, a transplant recipient suddenly finds himself able to live a full life. Organ recipients can work, they can travel, they can play with their children or grandchildren, and they can enjoy everything that life has to offer. On the other hand, it's also important to remember that transplant surgery involves many risks, that living with a transplant can be quite challenging, and that outcomes are often imperfect.

In this chapter, we'll first present some of the critical data about organ transplants in the United States. Then we'll discuss how to decide whether organ transplant is a good option for you, and if so, where you should get your transplant done. Next we'll discuss how to learn more about transplants.

Because some people are confused by moral and philosophical questions about transplants, we'll look at what various religions teach about organ transplantation. Finally, we'll debunk some of the pervasive myths surrounding organ transplantation.

A word about terminology

Sometimes it seems that people in the transplant field speak a language all their own. We'll define most unfamiliar words as they are needed in this book, but for now here are some of the most common terms used in transplantation:

- **Cadaveric donor.** Cadaveric donors are people who have been declared dead. Their families (who are often called *donor families*) consent to have their organs removed.

- **Donor.** The person who donates the organ.

- **Graft.** The transplanted organ.

- **Harvest.** To remove the organ from the donor. While some people in the transplant field continue to use this term, it's considered insensitive by most. Preferred alternatives include *recover*, *procure*, and *retrieve*.

- **Living donor.** Living donors consent to have an organ they can live without—such as one of their two kidneys or a piece of their liver— removed. Living donors are further subdivided into *living related donors*, who are blood relatives of the recipient, and *living unrelated donors* (including spouses), who are not blood relatives.

- **Recipient.** The person who acquires a new organ.

- **Rejection.** Rejection is what happens when the recipient's immune system attacks a transplanted organ. *Anti-rejection* or *immunosuppressive* drugs combat rejection.

- **Solid-organ transplants.** Solid-organ transplants include heart, lung, liver, kidney, pancreas, and intestine.

- **Tissue transplants.** Tissue transplants include corneas, skin, bone, and bone marrow.

- **Tx.** A common abbreviation for the word "transplant."

Critical data

Successful organ transplants are a fairly recent development in medical science. Dr. Joseph E. Murray of Brigham and Women's Hospital in Boston performed the first successful kidney transplant—between identical twins—in 1954. Dr. Thomas Starzl performed the first successful liver transplant at the University of Colorado in 1967. Within weeks of each other, in December 1967 and January 1968, Dr. Christiaan Barnard of South Africa and Dr. Norman Shumway of Stanford University performed the first successful heart transplants.

While surgeons continued to refine their techniques through the 1970s, serious problems with organ rejection prevented transplants from becoming widespread. But then, in the early 1980s, several new anti-rejection drugs—most notably cyclosporine—became available, and suddenly transplant recipients could expect to have their grafts survive for years or even decades.

The development of truly effective immunosuppressive drugs has been directly responsible for today's routine use and widespread availability of organ transplantation. In the period from 1988 to 1998, for example, the annual number of solid-organ transplants increased from 12,789 to 21,926—71 percent.[1]

The main reason doctors perform so many transplants is that experience shows that transplants work. Transplant recipients are surviving to live long and satisfying lives. In a study of patients receiving transplants between 1987 and 1995, the United Network for Organ Sharing (UNOS) found that 84.8 percent of the kidney recipients, 82.7 percent of the pancreas recipients, 71.8 percent of the liver recipients, 71.7 percent of the heart recipients, and 48.8 percent of the lung recipients had survived four years or more. These figures certainly underestimate the survival rates of patients transplanted today, since physicians have improved their techniques a great deal in the last dozen or so years.

Since transplants now work so well, more and more people are becoming eligible for these life-saving procedures. At the end of 1988, a total of 16,026 people were on the list for solid-organ transplants in the US. By the end of 1998, that number had mushroomed to 64,423, an increase of 302 percent.

Unfortunately, the number of organ donors, living and cadaveric, has not kept pace with the rapidly increasing number of people who are listed for transcript. In 1988, there was a total of 5,906 organ donors (1,826 living and 4,080 cadaveric), and by 1998 that number had grown to 9,913 (4,122 living and 5,791 cadaveric), an increase of just 68 percent. (The number of donors in a given year is always much lower than the number of transplants, since a single cadaveric donor can be the source of several life-saving organs.)

For the most up-to-date data on organ transplantation, see the UNOS web site at *http://www.unos.org/*.

Deciding on transplant

If your doctor says that she thinks you might need a transplant, the first thing you should do is to get a second opinion. Many people are reluctant to do this for fear of hurting their doctor's feelings, but doctors expect to have their judgements questioned and checked, especially when their recommended course of action is as drastic as a transplant. Most insurance companies and managed care organizations will pay for second opinions.

Even if the second opinion agrees with the first, and both recommend transplant, it doesn't mean that you must get one. You are an autonomous individual, and you have the power to make your own decisions about medical care. You should make this decision deliberately and only after you're in full possession of the facts. Don't be afraid to ask lots of questions of your doctor and other members of the transplant team. An excellent book about dealing with medical professionals is *Working with Your Doctor: Getting the Healthcare You Deserve*, by Nancy Keene (also published by O'Reilly).

For many people, the decision to undergo a transplant seems to be an easy one. When your doctor tells you a transplant is your only hope of avoiding death from liver, kidney, lung, or heart disease (for example), your first instinct will probably be to say, reflexively, "Go for it."

But you need to remember that while transplants may be routine to the doctors who perform these operations, transplants involve major surgery, and you may experience surgical complications, postoperative pain, and a difficult recovery period. In addition, unless you're receiving a transplant from an identical twin, you're going to be tethered to the medical system for the rest of your life. Organ rejection is an ever-present possibility, so you'll be taking powerful immunosuppressive drugs that leave you open to the risk of infection and other serious side effects, including cancer. In addition, the transplant itself and the lifetime regimen of immunosuppressive drugs may present a formidable—and continuing—financial burden.

James Theodore, MD, a pulmonologist at Stanford University Medical Center, explains that prospective transplant patients must be absolutely certain that they have the fortitude to bear these burdens:

> I think that the patient has to decide what the quality of their life is and whether they're going to be totally committed to meeting a fairly rigorous regimen. Don't do it because someone else tells you to do it. A lot of people want to live, but they're not too anxious to push themselves hard enough.
>
> I tell patients that they have to be 125 percent sure. If they're only 75 percent sure and say, "Well, I have no other choice," I tell them, "That's not good enough, because when you run into difficult times, that's when you'll quit and say you don't care." People give up on themselves and they die. So they have to feel totally committed to follow a very rigorous regimen with total discipline and total dedication. They have to get themselves physically fit and maintain that fitness afterwards. That's the ideal.

Double-lung recipient Kathryn M. Flynn thinks that, harsh as it may seem, it's right for medical professionals to stress the high level of commitment required of transplant patients:

> A big thing they like to tell you in lung clinic is, "We're not curing you. You're trading one disease for another." And I used to be kind of angry at them for stressing that, until I saw so many of my friends have a lot of trouble with the transplant, and some of them die after one or two years. You are trading one disease for another, and the question that comes to mind for many people is, "Well, then, is it worth it? Is my new disease better than the old disease?" My answer is yes, definitely.

Kidney recipient Dave Souza agonized for some time about whether to go for a transplant. Like many kidney patients, he knew that he had the luxury of saying no to transplant while still maintaining himself indefinitely on dialysis. On the other hand, dialysis presents many problems of its own. Here he describes how he weighed the pros and cons of transplant:

> One of the cons of the transplant was taking pills that would lower my immune system, that could subject me to cancer and other diseases that I couldn't fight off.

And then, of course, there was the fear of an operation. Except for when they implanted the catheter for peritoneal dialysis, I've never had any other operation or hospital time in my life. I tried to just ignore the fear part and then weigh the pluses and minuses. Fear can make you make the wrong decision every time.

In hindsight, I've had worse visits to the dentist than this whole transplant experience.

Liver recipient Steven W. Rahn found that his transplant made a much bigger difference in his life than he expected:

I was in poor health clinically for probably five or six years, but I really was probably not 100 percent [healthy] since my mid-teens. While I always thought I was in pretty good health, after the transplant I really found out what good health was. It was startling to see the difference.

These kinds of transformations are common, and psychiatrist Kathy L. Coffman, MD, of St. Vincent Medical Center in Los Angeles, explains that it's one of the main reasons she has chosen to specialize in working with organ recipients:

I think it's very exciting to see the transformation. The patients come in and are very ill, especially the liver- and heart-transplant patients. After the transplant they have a good quality of life, and they have a lot of fun. It's a wonderful thing to be part of that—to see people literally brought back to life. It's kind of like specializing in obstetrics. Most of the time it's happy stories.

Choosing a transplant team

If you've decided to pursue transplant, your next step will be to choose a transplant team. Most likely your doctor has recommended one, probably at a hospital in your area with which she's affiliated. That's a good place to start, but you may also want to consider other transplant teams in the area or even in more distant locations.

The UNOS web site has a number of resources to help you choose a transplant team. You'll find most of these resources in a special section for patients UNOS has set up at *http://www.unos.org/patients/*. First, you should identify the transplant centers performing the type of transplant you need.

Then, using data from the UNOS web site and information you gather from your physicians and other sources, consider:

- The number of transplants the team has done.

- The survival rates.

- The average waiting times.

- The transplant team's "turn-down" percentage. This is the percentage of potential recipients the team chooses not to list for transplant. Small programs that lack a commitment to transplantation sometimes have high turn-down percentages. A low turn-down percentage is an indication of an aggressive team that may be willing to accept lower-quality organs than other teams are.

- The location of the hospital.

- Whether your health insurance or managed care plan will cover a transplant at that hospital.

- The support systems you will have in that area.

- Your general feeling about the hospital and its transplant team.

Some of this data can be misleading. You shouldn't necessarily focus only on transplant teams whose patients have long survival times, for example. Sometimes the best teams take on the most difficult cases, and those lower the overall survival statistics. Also, waiting times are historical in nature, and may not reflect how long patients enrolling now will have to wait.

Learning about transplants

As explained above, it's important to take an active role in managing your health both before and after transplant. The first step in that process is to arm yourself with knowledge. You'll find a lot of information about transplants in this book, but there are many other sources of information as well, and you would do well to seek them out. We'll list some of these in this section; for full contact information, see the appendix, *Resources*.

It's not enough to just read a bunch of reference materials in a single sitting or to listen to a single lecture by a member of the transplant team. The issues surrounding organ transplant are many and varied, and some of them are highly complex. You would do well to read and reread relevant sections of this book and to continue to ask questions through all the stages of your journey.

Nurse Joan Miller, a transplant coordinator in the Department of Cardiothoracic Surgery at Stanford University Medical Center, points out that in her experience it's all too easy for transplant patients to forget crucial information:

> By and large, I found that even though patients will tell you after transplant that they wish they had known more before transplant, my experience is that even when you tell them, they don't remember. Before the transplant, they really don't much care how the drugs might affect them, or that they might have to have heart biopsies, and so on. They're focused on only one thing and that's living, and they will say yes to just about anything.
>
> Later, when they're feeling better and they're dealing with some of the side effects of drugs or the tedium of lifetime medical commitments, they will say, "If I had only known this before." And I think, "Well, what? What would you have done differently?" There are very few people who would change their minds.
>
> It's often the same for family members—they just want their father, husband, brother, or sister to get well, and they want to do everything they can to maximize the potential that that will happen. After surgery, they also often don't remember more than 50 percent of what they've been told, even when they've been given written information.
>
> I've been in the pre-transplant clinic. I've sat with the cardiologists when they've gone over what I would refer to as the routine drill: "This is our program, this is what we do, this is the up side, this is the down side." One of the potential side effects of immunosuppression is an increased risk of malignancy. And time and time again people will say, "Nobody told me that before my surgery." And I think, "Well, I'm sure they did." I've heard it too many times when I was there to think it would ever be left out just those times I happened to be out of the room. "Well, nobody told me that these drugs might damage my kidneys." Yes, they did. These side effects don't happen to everybody, and you don't want it to happen to yourself. So you don't hear, and you don't remember.

Educating yourself about transplants must be a continuous and ongoing process. Fortunately, there is a wealth of resources—in bookstores, libraries, on the Internet, and elsewhere—that can provide a steady stream of information about every detail of the transplant experience.

Some people believe that they'll be unable to understand all this information since they have no background in medicine. But in fact, if you're reasonably intelligent, you can easily educate yourself in one narrow area of medical science.

You should start small, by reading every piece of patient-education material you can get your hands on. Gradually you'll find yourself able to understand more technical material.

It'll help if you can get your hands on a comprehensive medical dictionary. We recommend Clayton L. Thomas (Editor), *Taber's Cyclopedic Medical Dictionary* (Philadelphia: F.A. Davis Co., 1997), since it's geared toward the nursing profession and tends to have a good deal of practical information that other dictionaries lack. Other good medical dictionaries are: Thomas Lathrop Stedman, *Stedman's Medical Dictionary* (Williams & Wilkins, 1995), and W. A. Newman Dorland (Editor), *Dorland's Illustrated Medical Dictionary* (W. B. Saunders Co., 1994). All three of these dictionaries are updated every few years, and you should always try to obtain the most recent edition.

UNOS maintains an excellent web site at *http://www.unos.org/* with a great deal of educational material geared toward patients. An even better site with even more information for transplant patients is called TransWeb: *http://www.transweb.org/*. TransWeb's "Question and Answer" section contains an especially thorough discussion of many of the common concerns of transplant patients.

Stadtlanders Pharmacy is a nationwide, mail-order pharmacy specializing in the needs of transplant patients. It publishes a very well-written magazine called *LifeTimes* that contains a wealth of information of interest to transplant patients. The pharmacy will send a free issue on request to anyone who asks, and if you choose to participate in any of its programs, you'll get a free subscription. Call (800) 238-7828 for more information, or visit the web site at *http://www.stadtlander.com/* where you'll find many informative articles from back issues of *LifeTimes*.

An email discussion group called TRNSPLNT, which is discussed more fully in Chapter 11, *Family and Support*, hosts ongoing discussions about transplants among many active and extremely knowledgeable participants, including recipients and physicians. For information about subscribing and retrieving archives of past discussions, see *http://www.concentric.net/~Holloway/*.

Mike Holloway, TRNSPLNT's moderator, has compiled a massive Frequently Asked Questions (FAQ) document that contains a huge amount of excellent information (and, in fact, is a source of much information in this book). You'll find the FAQ at *http://www.faqs.org/faqs/medicine/transplant-faq/part1/*.

A twice-monthly newsletter called *Transplant News* is the foremost source of information for professionals working in the transplant community. Transplant recipients too will find much of interest in its pages, but its subscription rate of more than $300 per year may put it out of reach. If you find yourself craving the same level of detail about developments in the world of transplant as a professional, you may want to see if your hospital's medical library has a subscription or if your physician or transplant coordinator would be willing to let you read some of his back issues. For more information, you'll find *Transplant News* online at *http://www.trannews.com/* or by phone at (800) 689-4262.

Transplant News also publishes the annual *International Transplant Directory*, which contains, among other things:

- A complete listing of every US organ, tissue, eye, and bone marrow transplant program, as well as patient support groups
- Listings of international transplant programs
- Contact information for all major transplant organizations
- Contact information for pharmaceutical and biotechnology companies involved in the transplant field
- Contact information for all US government agencies involved in directing transplant programs

You can order the current issue of the *International Transplant Directory* for a fairly pricey $99.95 (plus shipping and handling) by contacting *Transplant News*. However, if you don't mind using a slightly outdated copy, an affiliated organization called Transplant Awareness, Inc., sometimes has copies of the previous year's edition available for just the cost of shipping. To check availability, contact Transplant Awareness at the address listed in the appendix, or email *tai01@aol.com*.

Transplants and religion

Some people will question, on moral or religious grounds, whether they should be involved in an organ transplant. Just because a procedure is technically possible, it doesn't mean that it's moral or ethical. Virtually all major religions permit organ donation and transplant, some encourage it, and, for a few, donation is considered an actual obligation. Below is a brief summary of the teachings of many world religions regarding transplantation and donation.[2]

You should note, though, that in many cases these summaries render in just a short phrase religious teachings that may be subtle and highly nuanced. If you have any questions about the teachings of your religion in these matters, please consult a member of the clergy for guidance.

- **Amish.** Transplantation is acceptable if it's for the welfare of the recipient. Donation would be acceptable if a positive outcome was likely, and unacceptable if the outcome was known to be questionable.

- **Baha'i.** Transplantation and donation are acceptable.

- **Baptist.** Transplantation is acceptable and donation is an individual decision.

- **Buddhism.** Transplantation and donation are matters of individual conscience. However, there are many traditions within Buddhism, and some require elaborate rituals after death that could preclude donation.

- **Christian Science.** Transplantation and donation are individual decisions. Although Christian Scientists prefer to rely on spiritual rather than medical means of healing, individuals are free to choose whatever medical treatments they desire.

- **Church of Jesus Christ of Latter-day Saints (Mormon).** Transplantation and donation are individual decisions.

- **Episcopal Church.** Transplantation is acceptable only when needed. Donation is encouraged, but the ultimate disposal of body parts should be done reverently.

- **Evangelical Covenant Church.** Transplantation and donation are acceptable, and members are encouraged to sign and carry organ donor cards.

- **Greek Orthodox Church.** Transplantation is acceptable. Donation is acceptable only if the organs are used for transplants, not if they are used for research or experimentation.

- **Gypsies.** The Gypsies are a set of ethnic groups that do not have an exclusive religion. In general, however, Gypsies are opposed to both transplantation and donation.

- **Hinduism.** Transplantation and donation are acceptable.

- **Islam.** Transplantation is acceptable. While the Moslem Religious Council initially opposed donation, it has now reversed its position but requires that donated organs be transplanted immediately and not stored in organ banks.

- **Jehovah's Witnesses.** Transplantation and donation may be acceptable; however, all organs must be completely drained of blood before transplantation.

- **Judaism.** Transplantation and donation are acceptable, and in fact, if one is in a position to donate an organ to save a life, there is a moral obligation to do so. On the other hand, some branches of Judaism, such as Hasidism, may be reluctant to permit donation, regarding it as defilement of the dead.

- **Protestant denominations.** Because of the wide variety of Protestant denominations, it's hard to generalize, but for most transplantation is acceptable and donation is a matter of individual decision.

- **Religious Society of Friends (Quakers).** Transplantation and donation are acceptable.

- **Roman Catholic Church.** Transplantation and donation are acceptable.

- **Unitarian Universalist.** Transplantation and donation are acceptable.

- **United Methodist Church.** Transplantation and donation are acceptable.

Even when a religion has no specific prohibition against donation or transplant, there are sometimes cultural barriers to the practice. In Japanese society, for example, cultural taboos have long prohibited organ transplantation even though Buddhism, Japan's dominant religion, does not prohibit it. Japanese tradition requires the performance of lengthy rituals before an individual is regarded as having passed on, and by the time the rituals are complete, most organs are not suitable for transplant. But the taboo against transplant and donation seems to be easing, and in 1999, physicians began performing a few transplants in Japan.

Transplant myths

Quite a number of myths, rumors, and misconceptions have arisen regarding organ donation and transplantation. Such myths are almost always unfounded, but they all tend to make people less willing to donate their organs or the organs of a loved one who has just died. Here, in no particular order, is the real scoop on some of the most common myths.

Myth: Cadaveric donors may not really be dead

Many people worry that if they allow their organs—or those of a loved one—to be donated, that the organs will be taken before the person is actually dead. It is true that doctors do not wait for the donor's heart to stop beating before procuring the organs. If they did, transplants would succeed much less frequently, since organs begin deteriorating rapidly when they're separated from their blood supply. For that reason, the best donor is a person whose brain has ceased all activity, but whose heart is still beating. This is sometimes referred to as "brain death," although some transplant professionals dislike the use of the term, preferring to call it, more simply and less confusingly, death.

You may have heard stories of people who have awakened from comas, but the truth is that brain death is entirely distinct from coma. Someone who is brain dead will have no detectable brain activity or blood flow in either higher or lower centers of the brain. Such a person cannot breathe unassisted, and experiences no thoughts or sensations. Unlike a coma or a "vegetative state," brain death is irreversible, and there has never been a clinically documented case of a person recovering after being declared brain dead. For someone to be declared brain dead, two physicians must confirm this at two separate times.

Myth: There is a black market in organs

The law in the United States, Canada, Mexico, and all of Europe specifically prohibits the sale of organs for transplant. Unfortunately, the law in India is more lax, and in some Indian cities, a poor person can make some money by selling one of his or her kidneys.

But there is no evidence that—as persistent urban legends have it—organs are routinely stolen from people who have been secretly drugged, only to wake up hours later with a surgical scar and a missing kidney. Procuring an organ from anyone—alive or dead—is a complex business, requiring a highly skilled surgical team and the facilities of a major hospital. It can't be done successfully in a back alley.

On top of that, the organ matching and distribution system is quite complex and well monitored, and it's difficult to see how stolen organs could possibly make their way into such a system. For a black market to be active, a large conspiracy of evil, powerful, and wealthy people would have had to set up a parallel matching and distribution system, including doctors, nurses, hospitals, and private organ procurement organizations. Even if someone were that evil, powerful, and wealthy, there'd be no point in going to all this trouble.

Related to this is the rumor that Latin American babies are routinely kidnapped, transported to the US, and used for their organs. These rumors apparently began in 1986 as part of a Soviet disinformation campaign. Despite the fact that these rumors are widely believed—even, apparently, by some government officials in Latin America—no one has ever presented the slightest evidence that any babies have ever been kidnapped for their organs.

Myth: Organs are allocated in a racist manner

It is true that African Americans tend to wait longer for organs, but racism is apparently not a direct cause. People are more likely to find a matching organ from within their own ethnic group. Unfortunately, African Americans tend to have higher rates of diabetes, kidney disease, and heart disease, leading to a greater need for organs.

Paradoxically, the very idea that organs are allocated in an unfair manner can have the effect of making things worse. If somebody believes that organ allocation is racist, he or she may be less willing to donate. This in turn decreases the chance that others who need transplants will find matching donors.

Myth: Wealthy or famous people receive preferential treatment

People are not listed by name in the national and regional transplant lists, so it would be difficult to treat anyone preferentially even if somebody wanted to do so.

This rumor may have arisen partly from the cases of baseball great Mickey Mantle and Pennsylvania governor Robert P. Casey, both of whom received transplants shortly after being placed on the list. An investigation by UNOS of the Mickey Mantle allegations revealed that, among people of the appropriate blood type, he was the sickest person in his region at the time a liver became available. In the case of Governor Casey, he needed both a heart and a liver, and in his region at that time, anyone who required a multi-organ transplant was put on the top of the list.

Some people worry that wealthy foreigners could come to the US and buy their way to the top of the transplant list, displacing Americans. In fact, any foreign person who qualifies for transplant (and has the resources to pay for it) can be placed on the US list, where they are given the same treatment as any American. Likewise, foreigners who die in the US are eligible to donate their organs here. UNOS has a policy that discourages US transplant centers from performing more than 10 percent of their transplants on non-citizens, and the actual percentages at most transplant centers are much lower.

Myth: Organ donation requires mutilation

In fact, surgeons take the utmost of care when removing organs from a cadaveric donor. Organ donation will not interfere with normal funeral arrangements.

Myth: Donor families must pay

In fact, it is the recipient (or more frequently, the recipient's medical plan) that pays for all costs surrounding organ donation. Donor families should contact the local organ procurement organization if they believe they have been billed improperly.

Myth: Potential donors get worse medical treatment

Some people believe that they'll get substandard medical care in an emergency situation if they've indicated a willingness to be an organ donor. In fact, the medical team treating you in an emergency is entirely separate from the organ procurement team. The organ procurement organization is called only after all life-saving efforts have failed and you have been declared dead.

Myth: Recipients might discover the donor's identity

Some people worry that the recipients may discover the donor's identity—or vice versa—and they worry that the other family may make demands or cause grief in other ways. Organ procurement organizations (OPOs) take steps to prevent that from happening. They will never give out names or contact information unless all parties consent. OPOs will, however, transmit anonymous letters between recipients and donor families.

Nevertheless, there is more than a grain of truth to this myth. There are other ways that recipients and donor families could possibly learn the other's identity, by accident or on purpose. For example, the news media might broadcast information about the car crash that is the cause of the donor's death and reveal the identity of a donor that way.

See Chapter 14, *Donors and Recipients*, for more information on the remarkable connections between these two groups of people.

Myth: If you're willing to donate, it's enough to sign a donor card

Of all the myths and misconceptions listed in this section, this one has the most dangerous effects. While everyone is encouraged to sign a donor card or to indicate their preferences on a driver's license and to carry it with them at all times, it's not enough. First of all, wallets sometimes become separated from their owners after an accident. More importantly, however, your family has the final say about the disposition of your organs in the event of your death. While in some jurisdictions your family may have a legal obligation to follow your wishes, in practice, hospitals and organ procurement organizations will follow the family's directives no matter what a piece of paper in your wallet may say. Your family may not even know of your desire to be an organ donor. In their grief, many families refuse even to consider organ donation.

The one way to encourage your family to respect your wishes regarding donation is to discuss it with them. Don't wait. Do it today. Share your decision with them. When the time comes, they're likely to remember that conversation and to follow your wishes.

The transplant community uses a slogan to capsulize this point: "Share Your Life. Share Your Decision."

CHAPTER 2

The System

IN THE EARLY DAYS OF TRANSPLANTS, individual hospitals—even individual physicians—managed everything, from evaluating recipients to procuring organs to maintaining a waiting list to matching donor organs with recipients. Few laws or regulations governed the system.

Nowadays, with more than 20,000 transplants performed every year in the US, such an informal system clearly wouldn't work. With more than 64,000 people awaiting transplant, there's a huge disparity between the number of donor organs and the number of people who need a transplant. Laws and regulations have been developed to manage the system as fairly as possible.

This chapter will discuss the organization and rules of the organ distribution systems in the US. We'll discuss the roles of the various members of the typical transplant team and how they go about screening candidates for transplant. We'll see how the national waiting list works, and we'll suggest several strategies that some people can use to shorten the waiting time. Finally, we'll see what happens immediately after you're listed.

This chapter deals exclusively with the system in the United States. Other countries have systems that differ in significant respects to the US system. Since the organization of the organ distribution system has such a profound effect on the individual recipient, we urge transplant candidates in other countries to educate themselves on their local systems, and not to assume that all or part of what follows applies to them.

UNOS

The United Network for Organ Sharing (UNOS) is the national organization that administers organ procurement and distribution. It will surprise many to learn that UNOS is not a governmental body. Instead, it is a private, non-profit corporation, located in Richmond, Virginia. The National Organ Transplant Act of 1984 mandated the creation of a national Organ Procurement and Transplantation Network (OPTN), and UNOS administers OPTN (as well as the US Scientific Registry on Organ Transplantation) under contract with the US Department of Health and Human Services. In technical accounting terms, the Internal Revenue Service classifies UNOS as a 501(c)(3) charitable organization.

UNOS maintains an extremely informative web site at *http://www.unos.org/*.

UNOS manages the list of patients awaiting organ transplant. Through its Organ Center, UNOS matches organ donors to waiting recipients 24 hours a day and 365 days a year. UNOS is also responsible for establishing policies to ensure that all patients have a fair chance at receiving the organ they need.

The members of UNOS include every transplant program, every organ procurement organization (OPO), and every tissue-typing laboratory in the United States. UNOS is managed by a board of directors, including among its 40 members medical professionals, transplant recipients, and donor family members. This board has final approval over policies governing the transplant community, which are initially developed by the UNOS membership through a series of regional meetings and national committees.

Organ procurement organizations

At this writing, there are 62 local organ procurement organizations (also called organ procurement associations—OPAs) organized into 11 regions in the United States. Most states are served by a single OPO, but some large states have more. California is served by five OPOs and Texas by three, for example.

OPOs form the primary link between potential cadaveric organ donors and transplant teams at individual hospitals. Each OPO's primary function is to coordinate organ and tissue recovery and distribution. Most OPOs also maintain extensive educational programs to inform health professionals and the public about transplantation and organ donation.

All OPOs in the US are accredited by the Association of Organ Procurement Organizations and are members of UNOS.

Until recently there was a three-tiered system of organ distribution in the US. With certain exceptions, when an OPO acquired an organ, it first checked with the hospitals in its local area to see if any patients awaiting transplant were a match. If none were, the OPO would check with other hospitals in its multi-state region. Only if there was no good match in the region would the organ be shared nationally.

As discussed more fully later in this chapter, this system has come under a great deal of criticism, and now at least some organs are shared nationally from the start.

The transplant team

Every hospital that performs transplants will have at least one transplant team. More frequently the hospital will have several teams, one for each type of organ transplanted. Here we describe the roles of the various members of the team. Some transplant teams will include all of these people, and others will include only some.

Transplant surgeon

The surgeon is the physician who will actually perform your transplant operation. He or she will take an active role in evaluating you for transplant when you're initially referred as a candidate. The surgeon will choose and monitor your medications, and will follow you closely both before and after transplant.

Other transplant physicians

In addition to the surgeon, you will likely be seen by another specialist in your condition as well. If you are a candidate for heart transplant, for example, you will be evaluated by a cardiologist. If you're a candidate for a lung transplant, you'll be seen by a pulmonologist, and if you're a candidate for a liver transplant, you'll be seen by a hepatologist.

Different transplant teams have different policies about which physician will be primarily responsible for managing your medical care. In some teams, the surgeon has the primary responsibility both before and after transplant. In other teams, one of the other specialists will be your primary physician. In still other teams, the cardiologist (for example) will be your primary physician before transplant, and that responsibility will shift to the surgeon during and immediately after your transplant. After surgical recovery the cardiologist will take over once again.

Transplant coordinator

While the surgeons and the other physicians get all the glory, the captain of the team is really the transplant coordinator, who is usually a registered nurse. The coordinator orchestrates every aspect of your transplant experience. The coordinator schedules the many tests you will have to undergo during the evaluation process, while waiting for an organ, and after the transplant. The coordinator gets the call when a potential donor organ becomes available, arranges the tests to see whether the organ is compatible, and sends a team to go and procure it. The coordinator is responsible for teaching you everything you need to know pre-transplant and post-transplant. The coordinator is the person you should first consult if you have any questions or problems.

Some transplant teams have several coordinators. For example, in the heart transplant team at Stanford University Medical Center, one coordinator is responsible for everything that happens up until the transplant, and others take over just as soon as you're wheeled into the operating room. Joan Miller, RN, currently serves as one of the team's post-transplant coordinators, but when she started in 1970 she was the sole coordinator, and in fact she was the first heart transplant coordinator in the United States.

Nurse Miller points out that one of the most important jobs of a transplant coordinator is being accessible to transplant patients whenever they have a question or a concern:

> We're the people patients can reach. They all have our home phone numbers. They can call us at night. They can call us on the weekend. I'm very grateful that none of them has abused that. I'm not officially on call at night and I'm not officially on call on the weekends, but if they have a problem and they're not sure what to do, we don't want them to be stressed or anxious. They can call and say, "Joan, what should I do?" I may say, "Go to the emergency room. This is serious. Move. Call an ambulance." Or I may say, "I really don't think this is a big deal. Calm down. Call me back in a few hours."

Not all transplant coordinators will give you their home numbers. Sometimes you'll be given a beeper number, and other times you'll be given the number of an on-call nurse. But there will always be someone you can reach 24 hours a day.

Nurse Miller continues:

> We do a lot of teaching when they first come to the clinic and when
> they leave the hospital. They call our office non-stop. And I tell them
> when they leave here and they go to New Jersey or Fresno or England
> that any time they have a question, any time they're not 100 percent sure,
> call me, just talk to me, run it by me. Five years from now if they hurt
> their ankle and go in to see an orthopedist and he puts them on a new
> medicine, call me and make sure that it's okay, because there are so many
> medicines that interact with the big immunosuppressants that they take,
> and we've had too many people get into crisis because of that.
>
> That's what I do. I'm accessible. They can call with anything at all
> that concerns them. If they have a fever, if they forgot their dose of medi-
> cine, if they don't know when to come to clinic, if they have a bad head-
> ache, or they threw up, anything out of the ordinary. I try to tell them that
> they have enough to be concerned about, that I don't want them to spend
> five minutes worrying about something that I could put their mind at ease
> about with a phone call. So I encourage them to call no matter what it is.
> If they're anxious about it, I want them to call me.

Nurse Miller points out that no concern is too small, since it's often difficult
for transplant patients or their families to know what may be trivial and
what may be critically important:

> Sometimes they'll just call with silly things. For example, they're sup-
> posed to take their cyclosporine twice a day, about twelve hours apart.
> "Joan, I was supposed to take my cyclosporine at 7 and it's 8 and I forgot
> to take it, am I going to be okay?" "Yeah, you're going to be okay." Or, "I
> can't remember if I made my clinic appointment tomorrow." "Don't worry,
> just show up. I'll make sure we have your records in clinic. It's okay." On
> the other hand, a wife might call and say, "You know, my husband just
> isn't with it this morning. He's forgetful." "Was he that way yesterday?"
> "No." "Take him to the emergency room, tell them that he's a transplant
> patient, that he has neurologic symptoms, and they'll call the surgeons."
> So it can run the gamut from the totally inconsequential to life threaten-
> ing. And they also know that if anything happens and they think it's seri-
> ous and medical, that they're not supposed to waste time with me. They're
> supposed to either go directly to the emergency room or pick up the phone
> and call 911.

Serious medical symptoms include confusion, irregular heart rate, shortness of breath, onset of pain, dizziness, high fever, anything that requires medical attention. With these symptoms they ought to get help sooner rather than later. One of the things I tell everybody when they go out the door is, "If you get sick on a Sunday night, if you've got a little bit of a cough and a little bit of a fever and you tell yourself, 'Well, I have a clinic appointment in the morning, I'll just wait and tell the doctors then,'" I say, "No, no, no, no! You go over to the emergency room Sunday night." Because I've seen people be at death's door by Monday morning with a pneumonia that just sort of blew into town and wiped them out. They're given a lot of leeway to come to the ER and/or call the doctors, and/or call us, because during the first two to three months after transplant anything can happen. I also tell them and their families that they are the last line of defense between themselves and disaster. They have to pay attention. They have to be aggressive, and they have to call when they have any question at all.

As the post-transplant coordinator, Nurse Miller has some special duties:

I make it possible for the doctors to continue to do their work, and the patients, with any luck, get the best care they possibly can, and yet everybody's lives keep moving along. I accept responsibility for patients from the time they go to the operating room to have their transplant. And I make sure that whatever protocols, policies, routines, agendas, or whatever my physicians want done on these patients, they get done. I review the operating room records. I'll go to the ICU a couple of times a week. I'll go through the chart and make sure all the orders have been written correctly and are being followed. We have a lot of residents and interns who pass through Stanford who are only here for a year or so, and they don't fully understand what sorts of protocols we use and why. They'll often discontinue orders because they don't think they are important, but I recognize they are. I'm sort of the caretaker.

Then when the patient gets ready to leave the hospital, my team is responsible for all the discharge teaching—getting him out of hospital, out to the outpatient setting. Do they need home care? Do they need to come to our ambulatory treatment center for IVs every day? Do they need a central line put in? Do they need their stitches out? Whatever they need, they call my office. All the paperwork that comes from around the country and the world, follow-up on patients, it comes to my office. I can answer 80 percent of the questions that come in. For the other 20 percent I can put my hands on a physician. If I have to, I call into the operating room and interrupt somebody and say, "I need an answer right this minute." I can wander around and find a cardiologist and say, "So and so in Kansas City . . . they just cranked their creatinine up to 3.5, and their doctor doesn't know what to do. I need to get back to them. What should we do?"

Floor or staff nurse

When you're in the hospital, you'll be attended by several nurses, who will deal with all your immediate medical needs. The floor nurse will serve as a liaison to other members of the team, carrying out the doctors' orders and reporting to them on your medical condition. He can also answer questions that you or your family may have.

Social worker

The social worker is the person who will help you with many of the non-medical issues surrounding transplant. It's the social worker who is often responsible for helping you deal with Medicare or with your insurance company, for example, although some teams designate a separate compensation specialist for this task. The social worker may also be able to help you arrange for lodging near the hospital and transportation.

One of the most important tasks of the social worker is to help you deal with the emotional aspects of transplant. If you're in need of counseling, the social worker will provide this service or will arrange for another professional to provide it. The social worker is usually the person who schedules and moderates support groups of transplant patients and their families.

Most social workers are highly trained professionals who have earned a master's degree in social work, an MSW. Social workers who undergo additional training and pass a rigorous exam can be licensed by the state to provide counseling services, earning the designation LCSW—licensed clinical social worker.

The social worker also plays a critical role in your initial evaluation for transplant (see "Screening" later in this chapter).

Dietician

Because of the specialized dietary needs of transplant patients—both before and after transplant—many transplant teams include registered clinical dieticians. Sometimes dieticians aren't formal members of the team, but are available for consultation when required.

Pharmacist

Transplant patients have specialized needs for medication not only after transplant, but before the transplant as well. Some transplant teams include a transplant pharmacist among their members. Whether or not a pharmacist is a formal member of the team, you should be aware that pharmacists are highly trained and do much more than merely count pills and put them into bottles. Often your pharmacist will be more knowledgeable than the physicians about a medication's side effects and proper use. If you're not sure whether to take a pill with meals or between meals, for example, be sure to ask the pharmacist. Also, be sure to consult the pharmacist if you're taking any herbal or "natural" remedies. Some of these contain very powerful substances that can interact with your other medications, and the pharmacist can be helpful in factoring in the effects of these products.

Physical therapist

The physical therapist (PT) is an expert on rehabilitation, and is the person who will recommend and help you implement exercise plans both before and after transplant. If you follow the PT's recommendations before surgery, you'll be in the best shape for recovery, and if you follow the PT's recommendations after surgery, you'll be up and around much quicker.

Psychiatrist or psychologist

Psychiatrists and psychologists tend to the emotional needs of transplant patients before and after surgery. A psychiatrist is a medical doctor and can prescribe medication if necessary. A psychologist typically has earned a PhD degree, but cannot prescribe medication. In the early days of transplant, one or the other was on every transplant team.

As transplant surgery becomes more routine, psychiatrists and psychologists are less frequently found as formal members of the transplant team. But this doesn't mean that transplant patients have little need for their services. As described in Chapter 10, *Emotional Responses*, the time surrounding transplant can involve great emotional turmoil for both the patient and his or her family. If there's no mental health professional on the transplant team, there will certainly be someone in the hospital who can be consulted if necessary. Don't be shy about requesting an appointment, either through the transplant coordinator or the social worker.

Team meetings

Transplant teams are true teams, with each member bringing his or her special expertise to the treatment of each patient. As Nurse Miller explains about her heart-transplant team, the core members typically meet once a week to discuss any current patients who have had significant medical developments:

> Once a week we sit down—people in cardiology, cardiac surgery, and pulmonary medicine. It's open to anybody who's interested in transplant, but it's primarily focused on the people who actually do the day-to-day care. Dieticians, physical therapists, and nurses from the hospital can come. At that meeting we review every patient who lifted above the baseline that week. Are they in the hospital? Have they had another surgery? Have they just been transplanted, and they are not discharged yet? The surgeons will keep everybody up to date on that patient's care. If they are an outpatient and they've come back into clinic and there's been a red flag, the cardiologist will mention that so that should the patient come in on a Saturday in crisis, the bulk of the team has heard about him and knows what's going on. Are there problems? Are we having trouble with drugs? Are we not getting blood levels back from the lab? Does somebody need to intervene? A lot of those things first come up in that meeting, and then someone will be assigned to take care of it.

Screening

If you're referred to a transplant team as a candidate for transplant, you can be expect to be evaluated in several ways. It won't surprise you to learn that your medical status will be checked very carefully. You'll be poked and prodded and subjected to many medical tests. The exact tests you'll undergo depend on which organ or organs you may need. We describe those tests in Chapter 4, *Heart and Lung Transplants*, Chapter 5, *Liver Transplants*, and Chapter 6, *Kidney and Pancreas Transplants*.

But it's not only your medical condition that must be assessed. Your "psychosocial" condition is equally important. Your psychosocial condition comprises a number of factors, including your mental state, your family situation, whether you are an obedient patient, and even your insurance coverage or ability to pay the high costs of transplant.

The interview

The transplant team's social worker takes the lead in assessing these psychosocial factors, so your meetings with the social worker are extremely important.

Michael Browning describes what happened when the social worker interviewed him and his wife to see whether his infant son would be listed for a heart transplant:

> You go to a social worker and they sort of evaluate your ability to handle this additional load. She asked about our marriage, and about our support, and our occupations, and what our jobs were like, and things like that, trying to evaluate our stability. That was traumatic for us. I was afraid they would find something that would keep them from wanting to list our son. But actually, during the interview with the social worker, it was really benign, and they listed him soon after that, probably that same day.

Social workers have varying ways of evaluating a candidate's suitability for transplant. Mary E. Burge, LCSW, of the heart transplant unit at Stanford University Medical Center, likes to observe candidates as they page through photo albums and watch a video illustrating the transplant process:

> I use sequential photo albums and a video with people that each one, hopefully, can relate to. I have a big variety of people of different ethnic backgrounds and ages and genders. I go through and explain what is going on in each stage using these pictures and see what they pick up on. I see if a patient starts worrying excessively about something like a scar or something fairly superficial, or if they recoil completely from the whole process, or if they say "Well, I don't want to do this, but this is what I have to do" and start kind of facing it head on.
>
> All of these kind of things are for the purpose of preparing them, teaching them about transplant, but there are also ways of informing myself about their reactions and their attitudes. Since I do similar things with each patient and family, I can tell what the variations are. Even

though it probably feels to them more like just education, to me it's also part of the assessment process.

None of these clues is an absolute red flag. It isn't as though if you behave a certain way, you can't have the transplant. It's just giving me a sense of whether they can face reality, deal with reality head on. I would worry about people who are unable to watch the video at all or who really just refuse to look at the photos or to listen to any discussion of what to expect. Sometimes that just means that it's too soon, and so I just leave it and come back. But people who absolutely insist on having their head in the sand usually are saying that this is something that they just don't want. Occasionally, someone just doesn't want it because they they've gone through too much already. Usually it's just so scary and overwhelming that if you leave it and come back to it another day, it doesn't seem so bad.

On the other hand, some people think that getting a brand new heart is going to fix everything else in their life. It'll fix their marriage and their sex life and their boss will simply love them and everything. Some people refuse to give up certain things that we're asking them to, such as using illicit drugs or excessive alcohol or tobacco or, in the case of a patient who has suicidal tendencies, refusing to give up a firearm. Nothing is absolute here because these are human beings and we're just working with them. It's not like a college's admissions policy: you're in or you're out. I'm looking for evidence of emotional stability and compliance and reasonable family support so that they have a good chance of being able to cope with the whole thing.

Rae Ann Hopkins Berry, LCSW, a social worker at Stanford's liver transplant unit, explains why the psychosocial evaluation is so important:

One of the things I explain to a patient is that we're not trying to decide if he deserves a transplant or if he's worthy of it. What I explain is that if we put somebody else's liver in the body, the body will attack it. So we have to do some very high-tech, complicated things to make a liver work, including giving very powerful medication that causes side-effects that the patient has to tolerate, especially right at first when the doses are very high. Right after transplant we change the drugs every day. We'll always be changing a patient's drugs the rest of his life, but less often the further out he goes after transplant.

When we're looking at a patient, we're trying to figure out two things: can this patient do this, and will this patient do this. Those aren't the same things. We look at every patient with the thought in the back of our heads: Is this the place to put one of these rare organs? Would it have a good chance of working based on what we know about the person? Is this someone who follows through with things he starts? Is he a rule follower, or is he the type of person who has never followed a rule in his life?

Compliance

Stanford cardiologist Randall Vagelos, MD, points out that it's important for candidates to demonstrate that they're willing to follow medical advice and that they have a solid family support system in place:

The psychosocial aspects involve both the patient and the support structure. If the patient has been a non-believer in Western medicine, or is non-compliant with medicines, or is non-compliant with doctor's visits, or doesn't tolerate being in the hospital, those would really stand in the way of a successful post-transplant course. We assess this by talking with the referring doctors. If they call and say, "Mr. X is a great patient, he knows all his medicines, he comes to clinic all the time, and he watches his salt intake," that's the kind of thing we want to hear. On the other hand, if someone says, "Gee, I don't know how to reach this guy because he never leaves me his phone number, he doesn't keep appointments, and he never knows what his medicines are," we're less optimistic about his likelihood of thriving post-transplantation. We'll be frank with patients and tell them that. Often by following these patients in clinic before making these decisions, decisions about compliance and support systems become easier to make.

Ms. Burge remarks that during the evaluation, transplant teams are likely to take an especially close look at teenagers, who have a reputation for being lax in following medical advice:

As a group, the patients most likely to be non-compliant—to stop taking their medications—are teenagers. I think there are a couple reasons for that. Teenagers often feel invincible, that they're not going to die, that death happens to somebody else, not to them. Or they may have a transplant and do very well with taking their medications for a while, but then when they get to be older and less under parental supervision, they may start to do little experiments, by cutting their drugs down to three days a week instead of seven days a week, and nothing really bad seems to happen for a while. So they may decide to risk even more.

I think teenagers can often compartmentalize the different aspects of their lives and they can think, "Well, I want to live, I want to go to college, I want to get married. I want to play football, I want to do all these things, but I don't want to take these medications," and they sort of miss the connection in there. On top of that, some of the medications have a definite effect on appearance. The prednisone makes your face much rounder, and some of the drugs make you prone to acne, and some of them make you gain weight—all the things that teenagers are extremely self-conscious about to begin with.

Because transplant teams have a great deal of experience with non-compliant teenagers, teens (and their parents) should take special care during the evaluation interviews to demonstrate a high level of personal responsibility.

Support system

It's not enough for teens—or adults—merely to be personally responsible. As Dr. Vagelos explains, every transplant patient needs to have a solid support system to be considered a good candidate:

Part of it goes beyond the patients themselves. No one is a great transplant candidate without a support system—either friends or family who can be there when they are ill, bring them to clinic visits, bring them to the hospital when they get ill, and get their medications when they run out. But it's okay if your spouse works. That's the norm. They don't have to have someone who's holding their hand 24 hours a day.

Ms. Berry agrees that the support system is of paramount importance, so much so that she won't even conduct the initial interview unless the candidate brings along a family member or some other support person.

When a patient first comes to Stanford we set up an evaluation. Every patient sees me for an hour-and-a-half for an initial interview. I find out all kinds of things about that patient. I find out some personal things in an effort to determine how that patient has dealt with things in his life up until now, how well he copes, what kind of personal resources he has. I find out a lot about his support system: Who will be there to help him if he has a transplant? We really go into a lot of very personal detail. I also will not see the person alone. He has to bring a family member or a support person. It can be anyone who's close to him. If he shows up alone, I don't see him. We reschedule the appointment.

It is really hard to figure out a way to do a transplant for someone who has lived alone for many years, who has possibly never married, has no grown children, has either had no siblings or has alienated them all— people who are strictly alone in the world—because you cannot do this big surgery to someone and just discharge them from the hospital on their own. It is very difficult, but we work very hard to put together a support system who will help the patient. We have gotten people reunited with family members they hadn't seen in thirty years. It doesn't always take real well, but usually somebody comes forward to help.

Emmet B. Keeffe, MD, Medical Director of the Liver Transplant Program at Stanford, expands on the importance of having family support, especially in the weeks and months immediately after transplant:

The recovery from liver transplantation can sometimes be slow and complex, and you have to have somebody who can go shopping for you, who can help clean up your wound if you have a wound infection. If you're weak and you can't walk unassisted, you need someone who can help you walk as you begin to gain your strength back at home. You need someone to help you with all aspects of your living, especially during the initial several weeks after transplantation. You have to have someone who can be with you around the clock, not someone who is off and going to work during the day. You need a family support person.

Mary Burge points out that they are willing to entertain creative alternatives to the family support person when one isn't available:

Family can be defined loosely. Sometimes it's a friend or two friends working in shifts.

As we've seen, some transplant teams require that a transplant patient have 24-hour family support, while others are fine with spouses who go off to work during the day. In part this inconsistency reflects the varying preferences of transplant teams, but it also reflects the varying post-operative courses of different patients. Liver recipients tend to need a greater amount of post-operative care from family members than do kidney recipients, for example.

You'll find more about these matters in Chapter 11, *Family and Support*.

Alcohol and drug abuse

One thing that transplant teams won't compromise on is alcohol or drug abuse. If you are an active alcoholic or an active drug user, you simply will not be listed for transplant. Even cigarette smoking might disqualify you from certain transplants, especially heart and lung transplants. Dr. Vagelos explains:

> Almost all active substance abuse absolutely makes transplantation a non-issue. We think that level of irresponsibility is not compatible with successful transplantation. There are toxic interactions with the medications and both direct and indirect dangers to the new organ that alcohol, cocaine, or cigarette smoke create.

On the other hand, as Ms. Berry explains, past drug or alcohol abuse will not necessarily disqualify you:

> We try not to even interview the person or do the evaluation until they have been sober for six months. But even if they've been clean and sober for six months or more, we have the patients sign a contract promising never to drink alcohol again. That means no non-alcoholic beers, because even non-alcoholic beers have a small amount of alcohol. That means no Nyquil when they've got a cold, because Nyquil has alcohol. No alcohol means no alcohol for the rest of your life. A sick liver doesn't need to deal with it, nor does a transplanted liver need to deal with it. Also they agree to stop smoking because clean lungs will help them survive the surgery.

> We often require AA (Alcoholics Anonymous) attendance a certain number of times a week. We saw a man recently who was drinking up until recently, and we're requiring that he go to 90 meetings in 90 days, and then go once a week after that. Normally we wouldn't even list him before he was sober for some time, but this man is so critical that we're not going to have time to defer him, and we're sort of making an exception. If he doesn't start this and isn't going to the AA meetings, he won't get transplanted, but if he's into the process and doing it, he will be transplanted, and we'll expect him to continue the process after the transplant. All of this is individualized to the person, and their medical condition affects what you require them to do. But we require a lot. Most of the programs around the country use contracts like this.

Many of those contracts require the patient to agree to random drug or alcohol testing during the waiting period. The way this normally works is that the transplant center will phone the patient on a random day, and she'll be required to report to a local lab for a urine or blood test within a certain amount of time, usually two to four hours.

Transplant teams make no secret of their requirement for sobriety, but some patients just can't seem to take the hint, as Ms. Berry recalls:

> I saw a man about a month ago, and when I was asking about his alcohol history, I asked when he had his last drink, and he said, "Last night." I said, "Why did you do that? You knew you were coming here today and that you were supposed to be clean and sober." He and his friend looked at each other and he said, "We knew you were going to say that." He was expecting—maybe even sort of setting himself up—to be turned down.

Psychiatric evaluation

If the social worker or another member of the medical team suspects that a candidate may be suffering a psychological illness, such as major depression, the candidate will most likely be evaluated by a psychiatrist. But as psychiatrist Larry S. Goldman, MD, of the University of Chicago points out, psychiatric referrals are no longer the norm, and even someone suffering a psychiatric condition will not necessarily be disqualified from transplant:

> In the early days of transplant, the organs were so scarce and there was so much concern about only having the fittest candidates, that everybody was getting screened by a psychiatrist. But nowadays we have a pretty good sense that it's an unusual patient who isn't a good psychiatric candidate, although there are some. It's only when the medical or surgical team identifies a problem or has a concern that they'll ask for an evaluation.

> In the regular transplant situation, if you have a psychiatric screening and a patient realizes he might not get his liver if he "fails," then he presents his history in a more favorable way. So that's one of the many reasons that there has been a move to have less and less of the decision-making predicated on the psychiatric factors. The psychiatric factors are brought in more for treatment purposes or assistance rather than decision-making.

> *If somebody is depressed, you don't say, "You can't have a transplant," but you might say, "Let's treat the depression and see what we can do." Or if there's a personality problem, we might use either the psychiatrist or psychologist or a social worker to mediate between the medical team, the patient, and the family.*

You'll find more about these matters in Chapter 10.

The "green screen"

It may seem unfair, but part of the initial evaluation is a discussion of how you intend to pay for your transplant. This is sometimes called the "green screen" or the "wallet biopsy."

If you don't have health insurance or a managed-care plan that will pay, or if they won't pay enough, you'll have to demonstrate that you yourself can come up with the money for these extremely expensive procedures before you'll be listed. If you don't have adequate insurance, many hospitals will require a substantial cash deposit—maybe $50,000 or more—before they'll proceed.

Liver transplant surgery alone costs $150,000 to $300,000 even if you don't suffer any serious complications, and the cost can go much higher when you include medical care while you're waiting for an organ and while you're recovering from surgery. Even a relatively simple kidney transplant can end up costing close to $100,000 when those expenses are included. However, it should be noted that Medicare covers most kidney transplants under its end-stage renal disease program.

For more on financing transplant, see Chapter 15, *Financial Issues*.

Passing the screen

By now you surely realize that the transplant screening process can be one of the most critical events in your life. Pass the screen and you'll be on the list for a life-saving transplant. Fail it and you'll have to explore other options for managing your medical condition.

You have no control over the results of your medical tests, but you do have some control over how you present yourself during the psychosocial evaluation. You'll want to appear enthusiastic about the possibility of transplant. You'll want to convey your understanding of the difficult path that every transplant patient must follow, and your willingness to see that road to its end. You'll want to appear compliant with medical orders. If you've had problems with alcohol or drug abuse in the past, you'll want to be honest about it and firm in your commitment to remain sober. If you're suffering a psychiatric illness, you'll have to be willing to seek treatment.

But Ms. Burge says that during the interview with the social worker, you shouldn't try to be someone you're not:

> Be honest. Look the social worker in the eye. Be up front. Don't try to repackage yourself. Social workers don't go into this profession because they have a need to be judgmental, to play God. They go into it because they enjoy working with a huge variety of people, and in general a social worker is not one to give up on people. They're more likely to try to find a creative way to help somebody deal with whatever it is they have to deal with.

> If you have something in your past that you regret—drug addiction, for example—what social workers like is for you to say, "Yes, in the 1970s I did this and this and this. I stopped in 1986. I haven't done it since." Those people who can acknowledge their faults as well as their admirable qualities usually have a good chance of doing very well with transplants. Social workers are not going to say, "Oh, you were a bad boy. Nope, sorry, you don't deserve to live." That's not the point at all. As I see it—and I think other social workers would agree with me—none of us likes to turn anybody down.

Once all your medical tests and psychosocial evaluations have been completed, the transplant team will discuss your case. Joan Miller says that her team conducts those discussions right after the team's regular weekly meeting:

> After that meeting we have another much smaller meeting with only a core group of participants where potential recipients are presented— people who the cardiologists have been following, who they think may be ready to be put on the transplant list. They are then presented formally to the surgeons, who pick at every piece of data—"Are you sure this is right? Have you done this? Have you looked at that?"—to make sure that a patient is an appropriate candidate, and there really isn't anything else that you can do for him.

> At that time the decision is made. "No, she's not a candidate," or "She might be a candidate if you follow up on this and get more lab work," or "Yes, let's list her." It's pretty much by consensus. Sometimes the cardiologist

will really carry the flag for a patient. For example, the cardiologist might say, "He's a really nice guy, he's young, he's got a family," and so on. But the surgeons might reply, "He won't live through the surgery. He is not a good candidate," for whatever reason. And the surgeons have the final vote because they're the ones who take the patient into the operating room. It goes on their record if the patient dies in the OR. They have to account to the hospital, to the family, to everybody if the patient dies. So if they're going to accept the responsibility to do the surgery, they have to be convinced that this is a patient who will survive and will have a reasonable outcome. They have the final No vote, but we almost never get in a situation where it's not reasonably clear.

Now sometimes a surgeon will say, "Well, I just don't know," and a cardiologist will come back in a couple weeks and she'll say, "You had this concern, but we've addressed it," or "We've taken care of it," or "I called the liver people and they looked at the results of the liver issues that you were concerned about and they say it's okay."

There's at least one other way that the team's negative decision about listing a candidate for transplant can be converted into a positive one. If you need the type of transplant that can be satisfied by a living donor (such as a kidney transplant or some liver and lung transplants), you may be able to get a transplant even if you don't qualify to be listed for a cadaveric donor. Kidney surgeon Donald C. Dafoe of Stanford University Medical Center explains:

A living related transplant is the ideal situation because it's elective, they can be optimized for the surgery, they experience fewer rejections, and so on. So there are some patients who would not be cadaver candidates, or maybe they'd be marginal candidates, and having a donor will shift them over to the plus category at our center. Other centers have the opposite philosophy. They may regard someone as not a good enough candidate for a loved one to donate, but okay for a cadaver graft.

For more about this option, see Chapter 13, Living Donors.

The list

Once the team has decided that you're an acceptable candidate for a cadaveric transplant, the transplant coordinator will contact UNOS and formally place you on the list.

The UNOS list is highly complex and varies in detail from one organ to another. The heart and liver lists, for example, have elaborate criteria for listing patients as Status 1, Status 2, etc., depending on the severity of illness. The kidney list, on the other hand, places more weight on immunological match and the length of time a person has been waiting. In this section, we'll discuss what it means to be listed, and we'll briefly describe the lists for each organ.

It's important to note that your transplant team has no control over which patient gets offered an organ. When an organ becomes available, UNOS calls the team and offers it to a specific patient. If that team turns it down for that patient (for whatever reason), it goes to the next patient on the list, whether or not they're listed with that hospital.

As you might imagine, the details of the listing criteria are subject to a great deal of controversy, and policies change every so often. In fact, policies on both liver and heart allocation underwent significant changes during the first half of 1999, and there is every indication that these policies will continue to evolve. We'll discuss some of the most contentious issues later in this section. Finally we'll discuss two strategies that could possibly decrease your time on the waiting list.

The liver list

The waiting lists for people needing livers and hearts are heavily weighted toward the very sickest patients. As Dr. Keeffe recalls, these lists used to depend more on the length of time someone had been on the list than on how sick they were, and this had some negative consequences:

> As the organ shortage developed over the last number of years, doctors who are trying to do well by their patients figured that if they put patients on the waiting list early, then they would rise higher in priority and would have a better chance to get a transplant when the liver failure developed. But what has happened is that the list became clogged up with patients who are not in immediate need of transplantation. This has prevented patients who desperately need transplants from getting a liver because patients who simply have cirrhosis and are perfectly stable were filling up the list. In response, we developed criteria that said that to be on the transplant list you must have cirrhosis and signs of liver failure such that your life is threatened.

What I tell my patients is that we don't want to do the transplant too early, because there's a ten percent death rate, nor do we want to do it too late when you have far advanced liver failure, which jeopardizes your chance of a smooth recovery. Therefore, we like to optimize the timing as best we can.

People listed for liver transplants are classified as Status 1, Status 2A, Status 2B, and Status 3. (There is also a Status 7, reserved for patients who, for one reason or another, are considered temporarily unsuitable for transplant.)

While the criteria for classifying recipients are highly complex, in general Status 1 patients have liver failure with a sudden and severe onset, and are so ill that without a transplant death would be expected within a week. Status 2A patients have chronic liver failure, and are also expected to die within a week without a transplant. Status 2B and Status 3 patients both have serious liver disease, but their lives are not in as immediate danger as the higher-status patients. As a person's condition changes, his status can go up or down. The transplant coordinator is responsible for alerting UNOS to such changes.

The heart list

People on the heart list are classified as Status 1A, Status 1B, or Status 2. How a person is classified depends on technical medical criteria. Suffice it to say that Status 1A patients are the most in need of an organ, with Status 1B and Status 2 patients in somewhat less dire need. (As with the liver list, there is also a Status 7 that's reserved for patients who, for one reason or another, are considered temporarily unsuitable for transplant.)

The kidney list

As Dr. Dafoe explains, patients on the kidney list are generally not segregated according to the severity of their illness:

We don't have a staging for the kidney waiting list in the way that they do for livers or hearts. Unlike livers or hearts, where people are going to die if they don't get one of those grafts, we can maintain our people on dialysis. Kidney is first come, first served. When they come through our door, we put them on the list, and people wait in line. Occasionally, for a really extraordinary case, you can get someone priority. But it's rare.

The one exception to the first-come-first-served rule is the rare organ whose tissue type matches a patient perfectly. As explained in Chapter 3, a kidney that's perfectly matched to a specific recipient will be shared nationwide.

Lungs

There is no status classification for potential lung recipients. Donated lungs go first to local patients with the identical blood type as the donor, and then to local patients with compatible blood types. (See Chapter 3 for a discussion of identical and compatible blood types.) If no suitable recipients are found locally, the lungs will go to regional candidates with identical blood types, and then to regional candidates with compatible blood types. Body size compatibility and the length of time on the waiting list are also important considerations.

Pancreas

As with kidneys, there is no status classification for potential pancreas recipients, and the allocation is made primarily on the basis of waiting time and tissue type, first locally, then regionally, and then nationally.

National, regional, and local sharing

As described in the section on OPOs, earlier in this chapter, cadaveric organs have traditionally been shared first in an OPO's local area, then in its region, and only then nationally.

There were two main rationales for this system. The first rationale is based on biology. Organs deteriorate fairly rapidly after they are removed from the donor, and local transplants decrease the amount of time the organ is stored without a blood supply.

The second rationale for local donation is political or social. Organ procurement would be easier, it was reasoned, if people saw that organs were going to local recipients instead of being shipped away to some far-off state.

Whatever its rationale, the system seems to have resulted in some bizarre disparities. The waiting time for an organ can vary greatly depending on where in the country a person is listed. For example, according to an article in *The New York Times*, for patients with type O blood waiting for a liver transplant, the median waiting time in New York City is 511 days, while right across the Hudson River in northern New Jersey the waiting time is just 56 days. [1]

If you're awaiting transplant, it's important to remember that you shouldn't focus solely on waiting times. As Dr. Keeffe explains, there can be disadvantages to being listed in areas with shorter waiting times:

> The trade-off is that some areas with shorter waiting lists may have surgeons who are less experienced. If I were a patient, I would try to find the middle ground. I would try to find somewhere where I could get transplanted within a year by a surgeon who has at least a reasonable experience. I'd personally like to have a surgeon that has had at least one hundred and preferably two hundred transplants under his or her belt. There's no national listing of how many cases an individual surgeon may have done, but surgeons are honest. You could probably ask.

The policy of sharing organs within an OPO's own territory first before sharing them regionally has other odd effects aside from disparities in waiting times. For example, the cities of Dallas and Fort Worth, Texas, are just 30 miles apart—so close that they share an airport—but they are each served by a different OPO. One bizarre consequence of this is that an organ procured in Fort Worth is more likely to travel to Houston, 250 miles away, than it is to go to a patient in nearby Dallas.

Dr. Keeffe speaks for many in the transplant community when he says:

> I don't think that the current UNOS listing criteria should have such rigid geographic boundaries. There should be a broader area over which organs are allocated. How broad that should be, I don't know, but it certainly should be broader than local organ procurement organizations.

In recent years, scientists have developed methods that allow organs to be preserved much longer than in the past, making nationwide transport of most organs feasible and decreasing the persuasiveness of one of the two main rationales for local-first distribution schemes.

In March 1998 the US Department of Health and Human Services issued new regulations that directed UNOS to change its policy and to reduce these regional disparities in organ distribution. According to the new regulations, the sickest patients nationwide should have the first chance at any organ procured anywhere in the country.

Opponents of the new regulations—including many prominent transplant physicians and the management of UNOS—argued that they would have some highly detrimental effects. They contended, for example, that the new regulations would mean that fewer lives would be saved, since the sickest patients are more likely to suffer serious complications after transplants. An increasing number of those organs would inevitably go to patients who would die, and those precious organs would, in effect, be wasted.

In response to such concerns, the US Congress voted for a moratorium, preventing the new regulations from taking effect until October 1999 at the earliest.

At this writing, it's too soon to know whether the new regulations will ever be fully enacted. But in June 1999 UNOS announced a new policy for liver transplants that takes a step in the direction of wider sharing. Under the new policy, livers will first be offered to Status 1 patients within an OPO's local area, and then to Status 1 patients throughout the region. Previously, livers would go to other medically eligible local patients before being shared with Status 1 patients elsewhere.

There are excellent arguments on both sides of this controversy. In a sense, any tinkering with distribution policies is (to use a cliché) something like rearranging deck chairs on the Titanic. The distribution of any scarce resource, whether it's space in a lifeboat, or a special doll at Christmas time, or a life-saving organ, always engenders controversy. If a commodity is scarce, by definition some people will get what they need and some people won't. Any distribution scheme is certain to leave many people dissatisfied. As Dr. Keeffe notes:

> In the early days of transplantation it was "Can we do it?" and it centered on the technical aspects. Then it switched to the medical aspects—better immunosuppressive drugs, better control of infection, and some of the other medical aspects of transplantation. Now we're wrestling with some of the societal, financial, and political issues around transplantation so that we do what is best for patients in the US. We only have roughly 4,000 livers available each year, so our dilemma as transplant professionals is how can we optimize the outcome of those 4,000 livers while still being ethically fair to the individual patients that we care for. It's trying to strike that difficult balance.

No matter how fair a system is devised for the distribution of those 4,000 livers each year, it can never satisfy the majority of the 13,376 people (at last report) waiting for a liver. The same thing is true for hearts, kidneys, and other organs. The arguments about organ distribution will only stop when everyone who needs an organ can get one. Unless we as a society choose to drastically curtail the availability of transplants, this can come about in only two ways.

One way to address the disparity between the number of organs donated and the number of organs needed is by a huge increase in donation. In Chapter 14, *Donors and Recipients*, we discuss a number of proposals intended to address this issue. Unfortunately, all of those proposals have flaws.

The other way is to find alternatives to the use of human organs. Artificial organs or the use of animal organs for transplant are the two most widely discussed alternatives. You'll find more on that issue in Chapter 17, *The Future of Transplantation*.

Directed donation

One way for someone to jump directly to the head of the list is to have a donor family designate that specific individual as the recipient of one of their loved one's organs. If the organ matches, the designated recipient would receive it no matter where on the list he was. This is known as a directed donation, and it's explicitly permitted by UNOS's policies.

Donor families are not permitted to direct that the organs go only to certain groups of people. They may not say that only whites or only African Americans may receive the organs, for example. But it's okay for them to specify an individual.

Such a situation occurs only rarely. Typically it happens when the family of a person who has just died—and who is a suitable donor—happens to be acquainted with or related to someone who's awaiting transplant.

There's little chance that someone awaiting transplant could plan to take advantage of directed donation. For example, it would be unconscionable—and most likely futile—for a recipient or his family to wait around an emergency room, hoping to approach the bereaved family of an accident victim with a request for a directed organ donation.

While directed donation is not something you can plan for, it is something to keep in mind if a tragic accident does happen to a friend, relative, or acquaintance while you're on the list. Rather than approaching the family yourself, you may wish to consult your transplant coordinator for advice. Requesting an organ donation from a bereaved family requires great delicacy, and medical professionals with experience in this area have the best chance of success.

Multiple listing

If the waiting time at your transplant center is very long, you may wish to consider listing yourself at two or more transplant centers. UNOS rules explicitly permit multiple listing, but they also permit transplant centers to decline to list patients who are also listed elsewhere.

If you decide to try to be listed at a second transplant center, be prepared to undergo another full evaluation, starting from scratch. You may well have to undergo the same painful or uncomfortable tests at every place you hope to be listed. In addition, you should make sure that your insurance plan would cover the expenses of a second evaluation before proceeding. Many won't, and, as Dr. Keeffe explains, that's why wealthy people are more likely to be able to afford multiple listings:

> *Patients today are undergoing what is called multiple listing. If they have the financial wherewithal, they can go to regions of the country where it's known that the waiting list is considerably shorter and be listed at multiple programs. Some percentage of patients, usually those who are more well-to-do, have done that.*

Before you decide to pursue this option, make sure that patients at the second center are actually experiencing shorter waits than those at the first center. It would make little sense for you to be listed at another hospital in the same city, for example, since in all likelihood both hospitals would be served by the same Organ Procurement Organization, and would thus have very similar waiting times.

You also have to be prepared for lengthy travel at a moment's notice if you're listed at two centers that are not close together. Many centers require that their transplant patients be available within a specified time frame.

Dr. Dafoe points out that another argument against multiple listing is that the more distant transplant team becomes, in his words, "less invested" in someone who chooses to be listed at more than one center:

> *If you have the means and you wanted a kidney, there's no law against listing yourself in several places. That would optimize your chances. But it would waste a lot of people's time, and it's expensive. I personally think it's better to find a place, trust them, and go with them, preferably someplace close to your home. When someone does list them-selves in multiple places, and they end up getting transplanted in San Diego when they live near San Francisco, we as a center are not as invested in them if they get in trouble. We also don't have the advantage of knowing the person's medical course after transplant. That is, there's a lack of continuity. We'll of course do our best to take care of them, but it's better to identify a good local center, make sure they're good, and stick with them.*

Remember also the point made earlier that sometimes a shorter waiting time means a smaller transplant center with less-experienced surgeons. You'll have to decide for yourself whether that tradeoff is worth it.

Once you're listed

Once you're listed, the waiting begins. You'll find more on this difficult aspect of the transplant experience in Chapter 3. For now, we'll discuss a few of the things that happen immediately after you're listed.

Your transplant coordinator will make sure that she has good contact infor-mation for you. Give her every phone number at which she may be able to reach you—home, office, your parents' house, etc. In all likelihood you'll also be asked to carry a pager around with you. Sometimes that pager will be supplied by the transplant team, but if it's not, you should acquire one on your own. You certainly want to be reachable when that organ comes in, and you have no way of knowing whether that will happen tomorrow or not for a couple of years.

Kidney recipient Dave Souza was told that he'd be waiting two and a half to three and a half years for a kidney, but his beeper went off the first day he had it. As his wife Linda recalls:

> *We were celebrating my sister's 40th birthday. There were ten of us, and we took a limo to a Spanish restaurant in Larkspur. My sister said, "I*

keep hearing something," and it turned out to be Dave's beeper. When he went to use the phone, everyone in my family had a comment to make. My sister said, "On my birthday, it's going to happen." And then my father realized, "We don't have a car!" since we sent the limo away.

The beeper message turned out to be a false alarm, says Dave:

That number was only to be used by the hospital, although I did give it to a few people in case of emergency. But some nut-ball at work paged me just to tell me he wasn't coming in the next day.

Dave's experience suggests that you should reserve the pager only for that all-important call from the hospital. If you already carry a pager for business or personal use, you may wish to consider getting a second one—with an easily distinguishable beep—for use by the hospital. And since pager batteries frequently run down, be sure to check them at least once a week or so.

Some transplant teams may require that you be available within a specific time frame while waiting. This doesn't mean that you can't spend a weekend in Florida for your daughter's wedding, but if you do so, be sure to inform the transplant team of your plans, and be aware that you do run the risk of missing out on a certain donor organ if you can't get to the hospital quickly.

The most important thing to remember during the wait is that you should religiously follow all your medical requirements. As liver recipient Suzan Best puts it:

You should definitely do what the doctors say. If they say don't do something, don't do it. If they say do something, do it. That's one good way to stay on the list. You have to have a very positive attitude, and you have to be a strong person. When I was interviewed by the psychiatrist, I was told that they want strong people because they know that if the person is strong enough to get through other things in their life, then they will probably be strong enough to get through the transplant surgery.

Rae Ann Berry notes that even seemingly innocuous lapses can have drastic effects on someone awaiting transplant:

We tell our liver patients that they're permitted no illicit drugs and even no over-the-counter drugs unless they check it out with us. The things that a healthy liver can use out of the drugstore can be very bad for *someone with a diseased liver. Even aspirin would be a terrible thing for them to take. It could make them start bleeding and they might not stop.*

Remember that you're not necessarily home free once a transplant team puts you on the list. You can be taken off the list for a variety of reasons. Your condition may worsen to the point where a transplant would have little hope of succeeding, for example, which should provide a powerful incentive for you to do everything in your power to stay as healthy as possible. You can even be removed from the list if you fail to comply with your medical regimen, says Mary Waldmann Boucher, RN, a nurse in Stanford's Cardiac Advanced Therapy clinic:

> *The regimen that they have to follow in terms of medicines and medical follow-ups can be quite overwhelming, and if they aren't compliant pre-transplant, it's very difficult to imagine that they would be compliant post-transplant. That's something that we evaluate really closely.*

> *If they come to the clinic as they're scheduled, if they know their medicines, and they know the side effects, and if they refill their medicines appropriately, those are pretty good indications of compliance. The other big issue is their diet—the low-sodium diet. Some patients are very resistant to changing their diet, and they have a very hard time with it. Over a couple of months these patients really need to establish that they can follow the diet. That bares its head pretty quickly when they call up short of breath and we review what they've eaten over the course of the last day or two. If they've been to Kentucky Fried Chicken or McDonald's, then it's pretty clear where their shortness of breath is coming from.*

Hang tough through the wait. Trust that eventually the call will come. When she finally got the call, Suzan Best's liver disease had progressed to the point where her doctors were giving her only a few months of life at most without a transplant:

> *They said to be prepared because I could get a call any time, any day. We had already prepared that we would call up my parents and no matter what time it was, they would take us. They'd drop everything and take us to Stanford. We got called up around 11:30 p.m. on a Thursday. I felt scared, but also I felt relief. About two weeks before they called, I was wondering if they were ever going to call. It seemed like forever and I knew I was getting worse, so it was a relief.*

CHAPTER 3

The Wait

ONCE YOU'VE BEEN PLACED ON THE LIST for an organ transplant (as described in Chapter 2, *The System*), the most difficult part of the process begins: you wait until a matching organ becomes available.

If you are fortunate enough to have a living donor (a possibility for kidney transplants, some liver transplants, and—on an experimental basis—a few lung and pancreas transplants), your wait can be as short as a week or two.

If a living transplant is not a possibility for you, the wait can be as short as a day, or it can stretch on for months or even years. This can be agonizing for many potential recipients as their illness progresses. It's easy to become anxious and discouraged, especially since it's impossible to forget that many people die while awaiting transplant—an average of 13 people each day in the US in 1998.

You'll find suggestions for dealing with the emotional aspects of the wait in Chapter 10, *Emotional Responses*. This chapter will deal with some of the more practical aspects of the wait, including how donor organs are matched to recipients, and what you can do while waiting.

Finding a match

When you are a candidate for transplant, your medical team will carefully consider the best match between you and any potential organs, so you have the greatest chance of a successful transplant. To understand how donor organs are matched to recipients, you must learn a little bit about the immune system. The immune system normally protects our bodies from foreign invaders, such as bacteria and viruses, but it also has the unfortunate effect of making organ transplantation a challenge.

The immune system has a difficult job. We have trillions of cells in our bodies of thousands and thousands of different cell types, and among all those cells the immune system must find and destroy individual cells and viruses that don't belong, while avoiding attack on those that do belong.

All cells and viruses have a number of proteins floating on their surfaces. The first step in any immune response comes when the immune system recognizes cell-surface proteins that are foreign. Any protein that causes an immune response is called an antigen.

The immune system responds to foreign antigens in two main ways, called humoral immunity and cellular immunity. In humoral immunity, the B cells of the immune system produce a Y-shaped molecule called an antibody that fits into a foreign antigen like a key fits into a lock. Once an antibody latches on to an antigen on the surface of a foreign cell it neutralizes the invader in one of several ways. It can, for example, directly cause the cell to burst, or it can cause groups of foreign cells to clump together.

Cellular immunity involves the T cells of the immune system. Instead of producing antibodies, the T cells themselves attack and destroy foreign invaders. Receptors on the surface of T cells recognize foreign antigens, and then the T cells will either engulf the invader, or they will secrete chemicals called cytokines that in turn destroy the invader.

When foreign organs are rejected, the immune system is recognizing that the cell-surface antigens on the new organs do not match the body's own cell-surface antigens. There are two main sets of antigens that are of concern in this regard: blood-type (ABO) antigens, and tissue-type (HLA) antigens. We'll discuss each in turn in the following two sections.

Blood-type matching

Human beings have four main blood types: A, B, AB, and O. If you have type A blood, all your blood cells (and certain other tissues) contain the A antigen. If you have type B blood, your cells contain the B antigen. If you have type AB blood, your cells have both A and B antigens. Finally, if you have type O blood, your cells have neither A nor B antigens.

It is critically important in organ transplantation that donors and recipients have compatible blood types. If the recipient has type O blood, her body will produce antibodies to both A and B antigens. Therefore someone with type O can receive organs only from a donor with type O. But since someone with type O does not produce any blood-type antigens, she can donate organs to recipients of all blood types.

If the recipient has type A, on the other hand, her body will produce antibodies only to B antigens. Someone with type A can receive organs from another type A or from a type O. Someone with type A blood can donate organs to another type A or to a type AB. Table 3-1 summarizes blood-type compatibility.

Table 3-1. Blood-Type Compatibility

Blood Type	Percent of Population	Can Donate Organs To	Can Receive Organs From
O	47	O, A, B, AB	O
A	42	A, AB	O, A
B	8	B, AB	O, B
AB	3	AB	O, A, B, AB

Tissue-type matching

In addition to blood-type antigens, we all have tissue-type antigens, called human leukocyte antigens (HLA). There are three groups of HLA antigens that are important for transplantation. The groups are called HLA-A, HLA-B, and HLA-DR. Within each group there are numerous different antigens. There are 59 different HLA-A antigens, 118 different HLA-B antigens, and 124 different HLA-DR antigens.

You inherit one set of three HLA antigens (A, B, and DR) from your mother and another set from your father, for a total of six HLA antigens. A perfect HLA match is referred to as a six-of-six match. Considering the large number of HLA antigens, which can combine in an astronomical number of ways, it's rare to find a six-of-six match from a donor who is not a blood relative.

Fortunately, perfect HLA matches are not necessary in organ transplantation. Modern immunosuppressive drugs can prevent rejection even when there is no match whatsoever between donor and recipient in HLA type.

Nevertheless, tissue matching does count for something, says Dr. Randall E. Morris, Director of Transplantation Immunology and Research Professor of Cardiothoracic Surgery at Stanford University Medical Center:

> It's very hard to generalize, but broadly speaking, in the best possible world, it's always good to have a good HLA match between the donor and recipient.

But for a lot of organs, such as liver, lung, and heart, people are not selecting the donors based on HLA match, simply because there are not enough organs to go around. With kidneys, you can do that a little bit, but with lungs, livers, and hearts you don't have the luxury of time to ship the organs great distances. And also we found that with some of the newer drugs, the HLA matching is not as critical as it was years ago. But if I were a patient, and if I had my choice, I'd say, "Please get me a well-matched donor," because we know, even with new drugs, the better your match with your donor, the longer the survival time.

Figures supplied by UNOS back up Dr. Morris's assertion that higher levels of matching lead to longer survival times, but the difference is not overwhelming. For example, among living-donor kidney recipients with perfect six-of-six matches, 94.9 percent of recipients survived five years, while only 83.2 percent those receiving completely mismatched (zero-of-six) organs survived at least that long.

Donald C. Dafoe, MD, Director of Adult Kidney and Pancreas Transplant Programs at Stanford University Medical Center, notes that for some reason there's a much smaller difference between matched and mismatched organs when the transplant comes from a cadaveric donor than when it comes from a living-related donor:

HLA matching is not so important anymore in cadaveric kidney transplants. It once was thought to be the great hope. Twenty years ago people thought, "We'll match these kidneys, and they'll be accepted," because that's the experience in living relateds: a well-matched graft is quite different than a poorly matched graft. It's complicated, but that's not true in cadaverics. Nationally there are still points allocated for matching. In fact, perfect matches are shared nationwide. Eighteen percent of transplanted kidneys come from a national pool of cadaveric donors where the donor and recipient have no HLA incompatibilities. That's one way to jump to the head of the line. We could list someone today, and if they find a perfectly matched kidney in New York tomorrow, the patient has won the lottery, and they would have a one-day wait.

At Stanford, we actually give no weight to matching. That is for two reasons: one, the drugs are so good that the matching effect—though still there—is small, and two, when you match, you disadvantage minorities. Blacks already wait twice as long as whites. That's because whites are more likely to donate, but blacks are over-represented on the list because of higher rates of diabetes and hypertension. In California, we're ignoring a little biological effect in order to try to address the discrepancy. So, at Stanford, we think nothing of doing a zero-matched graft.

Dr. Dafoe thinks that there are more important things for recipients to consider than HLA matching:

> *Patients focus too much on matching. There are some people who say, "I'll only take a perfect match." We like to see patients taking charge of their own care, and we like to see them feisty—that's actually a positive survival characteristic—but I say without being sarcastic, "Which would you rather have, a kidney from a 70-year-old donor that's a perfect 6-out-of-6 match, that is flying to us from Florida, and that will have 36 hours of storage time, or a kidney from a local 18-year-old motorcycle victim that's only got 6 hours on it, but it's a 3-out-of-6 match?"*

> *I make the point to people that matching is not the whole story. There are a bunch of factors that need to be weighed in. But people focus on matching because a 6 out of 6 seems better than a 4 out of 6. Well, maybe it is, but it's only about 4 percentage points better. A young donor kidney is going to serve you much better than one from an aged and maybe hypertensive person. So, matching has some importance, but it's of limited importance. And the drugs are so good that they're beginning to completely negate the matching effect. This is our philosophy at Stanford. It varies at other programs. More conservative or less aggressive programs will wait longer. But I personally think that they are often penalizing the patient.*

While Dr. Dafoe says that matching is not that important for kidney or kidney-pancreas transplants, the story is somewhat different for transplants of the pancreas alone. He says that pancreas transplants do significantly better when there is an HLA-DR match, although HLA-A and HLA-B matches don't seem to be as important. If a potential pancreas donor does not have an HLA-DR match with the recipient, says Dr. Dafoe, "it's significant enough to be patient and wait."

Crossmatching

Even if donor and recipient have compatible ABO blood types and reasonably compatible HLA tissue types (taking into account that HLA matching is often not necessary), physicians must conduct a test called a crossmatch before determining whether a transplant is possible. In a crossmatch, a small amount of the prospective recipient's blood is mixed with white blood cells from the prospective donor. If the donor's cells die, there is said to be a positive crossmatch, the recipient is said to be "sensitized" to the donor, and that's bad. That means that the recipient's blood contains antibodies to some antigen in the donor's blood, which would cause the transplanted organ to be rejected immediately.

A recipient can be sensitized to a potential donor even if there's a perfect six-of-six HLA match. We noted earlier that there were three HLA groups that were especially important for transplantation, but there are a number of minor groups as well. If you are unfortunate enough to have developed antibodies to any mismatched HLA antigens—even the minor ones—the transplant cannot take place. (This may not be true for all liver transplants, for which crossmatching is often not necessary.)

A person develops antibodies only by being exposed to a certain antigen. If you have a positive crossmatch, how might that have happened? The three most common ways are by blood transfusion, by pregnancy, or by a previous organ transplant.

If you have ever received a blood transfusion or another blood product, you probably developed antibodies to HLA antigens in the donor's blood. If your organ donor has one of the same antigens as your previous blood donor, you will show a positive crossmatch.

Women who have given birth sometimes develop antibodies to some of their child's HLA antigens. This may seem odd until you recall that half of the child's antigens come from the father and are regarded by the mother's immune system as foreign, causing sensitization.

If you have had a previous transplant, you probably developed antibodies to any mismatched HLA antigens. If your second donor shares one of those antigens with the first, you'll have a positive crossmatch.

It's important to remember that while transfusions, pregnancy, and previous transplants can cause sensitization, they don't always do so. The experience of kidney-pancreas recipient Lori Noyes, while perhaps not typical, is at least not unusual:

I had a blood transfusion a year before the transplant when my kidneys were failing. So it surprises me that it was such an easy match because I thought the transfusion would have made me a difficult match.

Nevertheless, if you're waiting for a transplant, your doctor will think long and hard before giving you a transfusion or other blood product, for fear of sensitizing you to potential recipients.

While you're waiting for a transplant, you'll be tested periodically for your general level of sensitization. Your blood will be mixed with a panel of 60 different types of HLA. This is known as a percent reactive antibody (PRA) test. If your blood reacts with 30 of the 60 types, you have a PRA of 50 percent and your doctors would expect you to be sensitized to 50 percent of prospective donors. The test also tells your doctors exactly which HLA antigens you are sensitized to.

It's important to have a PRA test within seven to fourteen days after you receive a transfusion or any other blood products. In addition, since antibodies can sometimes come and go, many transplant teams will have you submit blood for PRA testing every month or so.

Other factors

In addition to blood type, tissue type, and crossmatches, there are several other factors that govern whether a particular donor organ may be suitable for a particular recipient. These factors include the organ's condition, its size in comparison to the recipient, the recipient's state of health, and the recipient's ability to get to the transplant center in a reasonable amount of time.

Regarding the organ's condition, transplant coordinator Lisa G. Levin, RN, MS, a nurse coordinator in the Department of Cardiothoracic Surgery at Stanford University Medical Center, explains that sometimes her team will decline an organ based on the results of medical tests or the donor's history:

An organ procurement agency may offer you a donor that isn't suitable for your criteria. For lung donors, for example, they may have oxygen levels that are less than optimal, or maybe they have a very heavy smoking history, or there may be any of a variety of things visible in the x-ray that would cause us to decline.

Size is also an important criterion. A heart from a 120-pound woman could not maintain the circulation of a 250-pound man. Conversely, a set of lungs from a large man would not be able to expand properly in the chest of a small woman. As Nurse Levin explains, some of these size discrepancies don't become obvious until the organ procurement agency calls with a prospective organ:

> We list our patients with UNOS in a twelve-inch height range, so even if I have a patient who is five feet tall, I'll be entertaining offers for her from donors up to six feet. While she wouldn't be appropriate for someone that tall, we want to make sure that we entertain all potential offers. They may not always be suitable, but they would come up on the list.

If the organ seems suitable for the recipient, Nurse Levin's next step is to make sure the recipient is suitable for the organ. One of the main things that could render a recipient temporarily unsuitable would be an infectious illness, such as bronchitis or the flu. Nurse Levin says that this is just about the first thing she asks when she calls a possible recipient:

> I say, "We have been offered an organ for you, and I'm calling to see how your health is today. Have you had any fevers? Are you bringing up any strange sputum? Have you had anything happening with your health in the last few days that we should know about?" If they say no, then I check with them to find out when was the last time they ate, and I make sure that they don't eat anything else.

> If the patient told me she had a fever, I would have the surgeon call her, because the surgeons would need to make a decision about whether we should bring her in or not. Fever really is not a good sign because the first thing we do is suppress her immune system, and if she has an active infection going then all you're really going to do is make it blossom.

Once she determines that the organ is suitable and the recipient has no infection, Nurse Levin determines whether the recipient can get to her medical center, which is in the San Francisco Bay area of northern California. Normally patients listed with Stanford live within an easy drive or a short flight of the hospital, but on occasion a particular recipient may be traveling, and could be disqualified for a particular organ if she happens to be too far away when it becomes available. Patients with plans to travel typically notify Stanford before leaving and become temporarily ineligible for transplant while away. Nurse Levin explains:

Next, I discuss with them how they are planning on getting to Stanford. The primary mode for our local patients is driving—and that's probably anyone within a three-hour driving window. But we do have access to Stanford Life Flight in the event that the surgeons are in a much bigger hurry to get someone here. We also have patients listed in all of the western United States. They can't rely on commercial travel, so they are required to prearrange charter travel, and we help them with those arrangements. It's really a collaborative process.

For more on this aspect of transplants, see Chapter 16, *Traveling for Treatment*.

The list

In Chapter 2, we discussed what it takes to be put on the waiting list for an organ, and we also described how the national, regional, and local lists work. Many people awaiting transplants understandably become quite concerned with their place on the list. "Am I in the top ten?" many wonder, and they rejoice if they've moved up to number five and become discouraged if they drop down to number twenty.

But for many reasons it's a mistake to become obsessed with your position on the list, and there are good reasons for thinking that the exact position is meaningless anyway. That's because organs are allocated on the basis of data, not on the basis of rank. You may be first on the list for a heart by virtue of having waited the longest in your region, but if the next heart that becomes available has the wrong blood type or is the wrong size, somebody further down on the list will get it. Since all donors and all candidates have all sorts of different characteristics, you may end up being third on the list for one organ, seventh on the list for the next one, and first on the list for the one after that. Even if you are first on the list, you might not get the organ if you have an infection or show a positive crossmatch. In addition, someone who's critically ill but is being listed for the first time can jump ahead of you if he is in greater need of an organ than you are.

Often it's difficult even to determine your position on the list. Most organ procurement organizations (OPOs) will not disclose this information directly to candidates. There are several reasons for this. For one thing, if they revealed your position on the list they might compromise the confidentiality of other patients. If you were told that you were number one, for example, you could be certain that the other fellow down the hall was not. In addition, your doctor may have placed you on temporarily inactive status—if you're traveling or if you're fighting an infection, for example. OPOs are reluctant to reveal this status information directly to the patient because they don't want to interfere in the doctor-patient relationship. Of course, if your doctor does decide to change your status, she should certainly discuss this matter with you directly.

If you're curious about your position on the list, your best course of action is to discuss this issue with your doctor or with other members of the transplant team. They may be able to tell you your approximate position on the list, but as mentioned before, you shouldn't focus too sharply on that number.

What to do while waiting

Joan Miller, RN, a transplant coordinator in the Department of Cardiothoracic Surgery at Stanford, says that it's very important for potential heart recipients—and by extension, all organ recipients—to stay as fit and as healthy as they possibly can while waiting. For heart patients, she says:

> What we do try to tell them is to be in as much control over their medical future as they can be—to be very vigilant about their diet, very vigilant about their sodium intake. They should be keeping their diet as absolutely good as possible so that their nutritional status is optimized. When you get into bad heart failure, you can start begin to develop muscle wasting, and if this gets too severe it could impact your ability to survive the surgery, and you might be taken off the transplant list.
>
> You also don't want them to gain too much weight. If they get too heavy, they'll never get a heart because they'll be too heavy for most hearts. . . to support their circulation. So they need to keep their total weight under control. Actually, a lot of patients have to go on diets to lose weight. A 250-pound man could wait three or four years for a heart big enough for him, because the bulk of our donors are younger and they're not 250 pounds.
>
> They also need to keep fluid off to reduce the load on their heart, and they do that by restricting sodium in their diet and by taking diuretics and medicines that help their heart beat more strongly and more efficiently. We focus pre-transplant on heart failure and how to manage it to keep them optimally prepared. They come to the Cardiac Advanced Therapies

clinic depending on how sick they are, either every week or once a month,
or sometimes they can be managed by their local doctor and just come to
us for checkups.

The waiting period is also an excellent time to have minor health problems seen to. Check to see that you're caught up on all your vaccinations. And be sure to get a thorough dental checkup. If you need dental work, it's much better to have it done before your transplant than after. Your dentist may find abscesses or gum infections that can be easily treated before transplant, but could turn into serious health problems if you waited until you were taking immunosuppressive medications.

When you're waiting, you should be especially vigilant about your health. Mary Waldmann Boucher, RN, and the other nurses in Stanford's Cardiac Advanced Therapy clinic urge patients undergoing evaluation—or already on the waiting list—to call with any problems or questions they might have. Among the problems that should generate a telephone call are shortness of breath, increased fatigue, or an increase in weight. The nurses evaluate the problems and refer the most serious ones to the cardiologists for further advice.

But Boucher says that some problems are so serious that you should not waste time trying to get her on the phone. Instead, these problems should trigger an immediate visit to the emergency room or even a call to 911. These emergent symptoms include severe dizziness, chest pain, or significant trouble breathing. This applies to all transplant patients, not just to those awaiting a heart.

Many heart and lung transplant patients are so ill that they must be hospitalized while awaiting transplant. The combination of a serious and debilitating disease, the strange surroundings of the hospital, and the anxiety-producing wait for an organ can make this a stressful and depressing time. While there are some suggestions about dealing with these issues in Chapters 10 and 11, for now read what Jim Gleason has to say about his experience while waiting for a heart. At first, he found all the changes disheartening:

> *Upon admission to the hospital, all the feeling of control, especially*
> *as I had carefully managed and understood my existing regimen of pills,*
> *was immediately lost. Pill schedules were totally different, medications*
> *were changed and their form was different (e.g., infusion replaced pills in*

some cases, needles supplemented still others). My first reaction to these changes was one of lying back and letting go of my responsibility. By day two, I was fast moving into a depressed state, a real detriment to the healing process. I asked my nurse, Mary, to help me regain control by making a list and schedule that I could use to manage my medication regimen again. She gladly supported this and even added notes on the purpose of each.

Sounds simple, but this was a major turning point in my active participation in the transplant preparation and as a key member of the team. Each day, I practiced and kept track of each pill delivered and taken. This was important training for the day when Jay, my wife, and I would return home and take on total responsibility for the lifetime regimen of pills. My philosophy was that there was only one member of the team on duty 24 hours per day, 7 days per week, with focus on only one patient: ME!

That focus, and Jim's remarkable will power, encouraged him to begin an exercise regimen in the hospital. He learned that a few weeks of complete bed rest can cause as much damage to muscles and bones as ten years of aging, and he was determined to prevent that from happening to him. If it seems unlikely that someone suffering congestive heart failure could stick to an exercise program, consider the fact that he enlisted two other fellows awaiting heart transplants as enthusiastic participants:

Obviously, while you are lying in bed waiting for a heart, there isn't much you can do in the way of exercise, right? No! Not true. There are any number of things you can do—and, in fact, must do—to increase your chances of success and improved quality of life post-transplant.

The transplant team encouraged any type of exercise as a way of strengthening the body for the upcoming transplant surgery. Not knowing how long the wait would be for the availability of a donor heart, you just couldn't lie back and wait. During my wait (which stretched out to five weeks of hospitalization), there were two other long-term patients—John and Ron awaiting hearts too. Both had already undergone long waits before my arrival, eventually waiting seven and nine weeks, respectively. John suggested we get a name for our little group and thus we became known as "The Three Heart BEATS" (for Bodies Eagerly Awaiting Transplant Surgery).

On any given day, I might be feeling lazy—ready to lay off the daily exercise—but Ron (who often did up to thirty-four miles of exercise-bike riding a day in his room—yes, while awaiting a replacement heart!) and John would show up at my door and announce that the BEATS were going for their daily walk, and so off I would go. What a sight, the three of us, each with IV pole in tow, John and I in colorful shorts (anything to get out of the drab hospital gown), walking (some days slower than others) around the exercise "track"—using that term loosely.

Our "track" was the hallway around the Cardiac Care Unit down past the Intensive Care Unit. With nothing to do on this walk, being a math teacher I counted the floor tiles, each measuring twelve inches, and thus calculated that once around the course was one-eighth of a mile. So, as we worked ourselves up over the weeks (yes, as the hearts were getting weaker, we were getting stronger through this exercise—both mentally and physically), we set goals of a mile a day (eight laps), quite an accomplishment in our condition. When mail would come, I would force myself to leave it on the table, allowing the treat of opening one piece with each lap completed (got to make this exercise fun).

Jim became expert on making boring exercise tolerable:

Another part of our program was education and support from a physical therapist. She monitored our in-room workouts using a bicycle pedal machine (an alternative was to use a real exercise bike, but that seat was tough to take). Again, the thought of time lost just exercising caused me to take my own approach, which involved something to focus my attention. This could be a TV show, or more often, a Walkman tape player with earphones to listen to music, self-improvement tapes, or even books on tape. While the therapist monitored heart rhythms, heart rate, and blood pressure, I would often be off someplace in my mind in another world based on the books I was listening to. Time flew when you were so entertained. When it came our turn for the transplant surgery, all three were in the best shape we could get in to improve our results. Finally, that time did come, for all three Heart BEATS in the same week! First Ron, then me, then John. Wow, talk about your miracles.

While waiting, it's quite possible that you may find yourself subjected to one or more false alarms, and it's important not to let yourself get discouraged by these. Melanie Horne had no fewer than five false alarms during a wait for her second pancreas transplant:

> With the first one, there was something wrong with the donor. The second one was a positive crossmatch. The third one, when they called they told me that I was second in line, and I may or may not be called for it. They just wanted to make sure I was in town and ready to go. They told me not to eat anything, and get ready because I might be called in. The fourth time, I was scrubbed, hooked up, plugged in and ready to go, and there was a three-inch-deep pile of nasty looking things they were about to inject into me, and then the resident walks in and says, "We found bacteria in your urine. You can go home now." But it turned out I didn't have an infection. The nurse accidentally contaminated the sample with E. coli. I was pretty upset. The fifth time was just last week. They called me at 7:45 in the morning and said, "Come on in. Let's get all your labs drawn, and we'll probably be taking you into surgery at 3:00." Well, when they harvested the pancreas it looked funny. There was some sort of weird anatomical anomaly. It just wasn't a textbook pancreas, and they're not about to take a chance with something that didn't look quite right. So we keep waiting.

One week after completing this interview, the sixth call proved to be the charm. Melanie received her second pancreas transplant, and as of this writing she's doing well.

It's common, as in Melanie's third false alarm, for hospitals to prepare a backup recipient in case the first recipient they call cannot receive the organ for one reason or another. Different hospitals and even different transplant teams within the same hospital have different policies on this. Some ask a backup recipient to come to the hospital. Some, as in Melanie's case, ask them to wait by the phone and not to eat, just in case they're needed. And some teams don't call backup recipients at all.

Joan Miller reports that in her experience backup recipients are frequently called when her team goes to retrieve a heart and both lungs (this is called a heart lung block) from a donor. The primary recipient will be someone scheduled for a combined heart-lung transplant, but other patients will be placed on standby. Nurse Miller explains:

> When we go out to procure the organs we're never 100 percent sure until we get there whether we're definitely going to take them. So if we've

gone out for a heart-lung block, then we may have a heart recipient on standby in case something's the matter with the lung, or we may have a single-lung recipient alerted in case something happens to one of the lungs and they can't use them both.

Sometimes the worst kind of waiting is the waiting you do after the wait seems to be over. You can be on the list for an organ for years and finally be called to the hospital for a transplant, but then you may end up cooling your heels for many awful hours before the surgeons are ready to begin. That's exactly what happened to Lori Noyes when she was called in the middle of the night and told to come in immediately for her kidney-pancreas transplant:

> *They called me at three in the morning said, "Can you get there at six?" I said, "Sure." I live about thirty miles east of the transplant center. My parents drove me in and I basically sat and waited. I have to admit I was getting pretty cranky about 2:00 in the afternoon. I said, "Somebody tell me something! Is this a go or not?" I was hungry, but they wouldn't let me eat. Finally, this wonderful doctor started coming in, and she would give me updates. She said, "It looks like you are the match." I said, "Well, aren't the organs getting really old by now?" I didn't know how else to put it. I said, "You call me at three in the morning, and now it's two in the afternoon. Aren't they getting too old to transplant?" Thank God, somebody finally realized I didn't know anything about transplants and said, "Oh, you don't understand. The donor is still on life support. The organs are still in him." Then I was at ease, because I was really getting worried about the time thing. They said, "The surgeon hasn't even driven out there to get them yet, because it's a little hospital and the donor has been put later on the surgery schedule. We deal with this all the time." My first thought was, "The poor heart transplant recipient is probably wondering what the heck is going on, because he's the one who's really on death's door waiting for this transplant. I'm still up and around."*

While the recipient waits, the donor team goes to retrieve the organs. Joan Miller describes the sequence of events going on behind the scenes when a potential donor organ becomes available:

> *We get a call from the California Transplant Donor Network (CTDN), which is based in San Francisco, and they are hooked up to the UNOS computer system. They identify donors, and then they call us and they say, "Joan, we have a heart for John Smith." And if John Smith has*

an infiltrate on his x-ray, or he's gone to Florida for his daughter's wedding, or he's got a fever, then we'll say, "Oh, gosh, he's on hold right this minute." Then they say, "Thank you very much," and they go to the next patient on the list.

If the potential recipient isn't on hold when we get the call, we then have them fax us about ten to fifteen pages of medical information on the donor. We look at the numbers: Is the echocardiogram okay? Are the blood cultures okay? We make sure everything looks good on paper. Then we tell CTDN, "Yes, we want the heart." In the meantime, we found out where the donor is—and also we've begun to call people at Stanford to say, "We have a potential donor run at such and such a time."

Often we get suggested times from CTDN. They'll say, "The kidneys are going to Los Angeles and the renal team is going to be there at 5:00. Can you meet them?" We always say yes. We always pull it together. If we're doing another case and our surgeons are in the operating room, we might say, "We can't send a team out for three hours, can they wait?" We agree with CTDN on a departure time from Stanford and a potential arrival time at the donor hospital, and then CTDN takes care of all the transportation. They get one of their technicians down to Stanford to meet our people in the emergency room. That person is responsible for all the technical support on the donor run and getting paperwork, getting blood from the donor, getting the solutions to pack the organs in, the ice, the cooler, all that. We get the team together and the surgical equipment that our surgeons need. Then everybody meets outside the emergency room and they go—depending on where the donor is—either by car, by chopper, or by fixed wing aircraft. It just depends on how far they have to go, and what the weather's like.

When they get to the donor hospital, our surgeons will go to the donor's bedside and review the chart, review the donor, look at the echocardiogram, and then take them to the operating room, and retrieve the heart.

Once the organ has been removed from its donor, it's rushed to the recipient's bedside for transplant, where the wait finally comes to an end.

CHAPTER 4

Heart and Lung Transplants

THIS CHAPTER DISCUSSES WHAT SORT OF PEOPLE will be considered for heart, lung, or heart-lung transplants, and it describes what happens before, during, and after surgery.

While the chapter focuses on issues specific to heart and lung recipients, it contains information of interest to the recipients of other transplants as well. Likewise, heart and lung recipients may find relevant material in Chapter 5, *Liver Transplants,* and Chapter 6, *Kidney and Pancreas Transplants.* Although the details of the transplant surgeries themselves are obviously different, all transplant patients, no matter what organ they receive, share a good many common experiences. This is particularly true of post-surgical experiences, and you will want to peruse those sections of all three chapters.

It's important to realize that different transplant teams have different ways of doing things. Depending on where you have your transplant done, some of the details presented in the following pages may vary. For a look at how one heart transplant team does it, you can take a virtual tour of the Temple University unit at *http://www.homestead.com/alouso/.*

Who gets heart transplants?

Almost everyone who needs a heart transplant suffers from heart failure, an inability of the heart to pump enough blood. Heart failure has several causes, including heart attack, prolonged high blood pressure, or cardiomyopathy, a disease of the heart muscle.

No matter what the cause, the result of heart failure is that a weakened heart muscle cannot pump blood efficiently, and blood flows more slowly through the heart. This can cause blood clots to form, and these can wreak havoc as they travel to various parts of the body and block blood vessels. If the clot blocks a vessel in the brain, the result is a stroke; if it blocks a vessel in the lung, the result is a pulmonary embolism; and if it blocks a vessel in the heart itself, the result is a heart attack. While cardiologists have an array of drugs they can use to increase the heart's pumping efficiency, the only cure for heart failure is a new heart.

People on the list for heart transplants differ from other transplant patients in that they can be so debilitated by their disease and in so much danger that they may have to remain in the hospital for weeks or months awaiting an organ.

Heart recipient Jim Gleason writes in his book *A Gift from the Heart* (available online in its entirety at *http://transweb.org/people/recips/experien/gleason/*) about the events that led to the determination that he needed a transplant:

> *Monday we saw our local cardiologist for swelling of the ankles —a sign the heart is not getting rid of fluid the way it should—and she confirmed the root of the problem. It seemed so long ago that the cardiomyopathy had led to pneumonia and congestive heart failure—but these were overcome in stride. This weakened heart of mine was now deteriorating further. The MUGA scan (an x-ray videotaping of the pumping heart) done Friday indicated it was now down from the 22 percent to only 15 percent effective pumping (versus a norm of 60 to 80 percent). The viral cardiomyopathy that resulted from a simple virus attacking the pumping muscle of the heart back in 1992 now showed signs that the aggressive drug program I was on just wasn't doing the trick any more.*
>
> *It was time to see the specialists down at the University of Pennsylvania for a possible heart transplant. Wow, do those words sound strange when you first hear them—and they were talking about me of all people. It was serious enough that the transplant team agreed to meet with us the very next day. It was recommended that I cease employment immediately—an action that was surprisingly easy to just do.*

Heart transplants are no longer the exotic rarity that they once were. In 1998, 2,340 people in the US received transplanted hearts.

Qualifying for a heart transplant

Not everyone with heart failure is a candidate for a heart transplant. If you're referred as a potential candidate for transplant, the transplant team will conduct a number of medical tests to ensure that you need a heart and that you'll be likely to survive the operation. Although some of the qualifying criteria can seem harsh in individual cases, transplant teams focus on what will work. They want to maximize the results from a precious and scarce resource—donated organs—and make sure that a life will be saved.

One thing to remember is that not all transplant teams use the same criteria. If one medical center decides that you are not a candidate for transplant, you may wish to investigate whether you may have access to other medical centers who use a somewhat different set of standards.

Randall Vagelos, MD, a cardiologist and Medical Director of Stanford University's Cardiac Care Unit, explains how his team evaluates potential heart-transplant recipients:

> *There are two issues that are important. One is whether in fact the patient is ill enough to be considered actively for a transplant. The second issue—which overlaps a little but is not the same—is whether the patient would be a good candidate for a transplant. It can be quite confusing to patients to think that they might be too ill for a transplant. In most patients' minds, the transplant is the last resort, and of course you could never be too sick to have one. But that's not the case at all. There are a lot of patients who are not good candidates because they're too ill or they have other medical or psychosocial limitations.*

(The psychosocial considerations that might disqualify someone from transplants are discussed in Chapter 2, *The System*.)

Dr. Vagelos says that of the 200 to 300 new patients evaluated in his unit every year, only 10 percent are eventually put on the transplant list. For one thing, upon evaluation the transplant team determines that some patients are really not sick enough to require a transplant:

> *I think the most classic example of that is the thirty-year-old who has been a very active alcoholic for five or ten years, in which complete abstinence from alcohol may allow some recovery—and possibly a dramatic amount of recovery—in heart-muscle function. To transplant someone without having factored in the possibility of improvement would be ridiculous.*

Dr. Vagelos says that some other patients are not healthy enough to survive a transplant:

There are some patients who have heart failure on the basis of a sys-temic illness, and this may be very important for the transplant candi-dacy, as well. There are patients who have scleroderma, for example, which is a mixed connective tissue disease that not only has a negative impact on heart-muscle function but also on the lungs, on the kidneys, and on the gastrointestinal tract. Identifying that systemic illness is criti-cal because the problems with the other organs would make transplanta-tion unsuccessful.

Other situations can also disqualify heart-failure patients, Dr. Vagelos notes:

Age is a big issue. Men in our society over sixty start to have prob-lems with prostate cancers, colon cancers, and they are starting to develop some problems with demineralization of their spine. Women at that age are starting to have problems with breast cancers and colon cancers and demineralization of the spine as well. People start developing peripheral vascular disease. Patients who have been smokers are starting to have lung cancers turn up. So that decade after sixty is medically active enough that patients who are older than sixty have to look biologically younger than sixty to qualify. We look for patients who as much as possi-ble have no evidence of end-organ pathology outside the heart. Diabetics, for example, often have kidney problems, peripheral neuropathies, prob-lems with their gastrointestinal tract, peripheral vascular disease, and so on. Those are all relative contraindications to transplant. There are also patients who have chronic lung problems, which would manifest them-selves as big obstacles for a successful transplant.

Almost no adult is too small, unless they are so thin that they are debilitated and weak. This can be a complication of severe heart failure. Patients who are over 200 pounds in practice will have such a long wait that transplantation is not really an active possibility, because you need an extra-large organ. Patients who are obese are not considered attrac-tive transplant candidates because one of the medicines that most people take after transplant—prednisone—has a tendency to put weight on peo-ple in a hurry. If they are already morbidly obese, we think the complica-tions of more of the same will make them non-competitive transplant candidates.

Many of these things in an individual's case wouldn't necessarily mean they couldn't survive a transplant, but they are very big obstacles.

*You're talking about a very limited resource. If you've got ten people wait-
ing and only two hearts, you want to make sure that everyone who's on
the active waiting list falls into a group that could maximally benefit from
the transplant.*

Mary Waldmann Boucher, RN, a nurse at the Stanford Cardiac Advanced
Therapy clinic, explains that it usually takes some time to establish whether
someone is a candidate for transplant:

*It probably takes two or three visits with quite a bit of testing to
determine whether or not they're a candidate. They may get referred for
the transplant evaluation, but their candidacy may take a couple of
months to establish. However, if they really are quite ill when they are
first referred they may get admitted, and then everything is done on an
inpatient basis. In that case, things happen quite a bit faster and they can
be evaluated within days.*

Many tests are performed to determine whether a person is a candidate for a
heart transplant. Although the exact tests you receive will depend on your
medical condition and on the preferences of the transplant team, these tests
may include:

- **Echocardiogram.** This is a test that measures the heart's squeezing ability. It uses sound waves to make an image of the beating heart. The test
  is non-invasive and takes about fifteen minutes.

- **Coronary angiogram.** This test is normally conducted only in patients
  who are old enough to have developed coronary artery disease—over 40
  in men and over 45 in women—and is intended to provide a picture of
  the blood vessels feeding the heart muscle. After injection of a local
  anesthetic, a doctor will insert a long, thin, and flexible tube through an
  artery in your arm or groin. She'll thread that tube through your blood
  system until it reaches the heart. Then she'll inject a dye into your heart
  to make the blood vessels stand out clearly. The dye may cause you to
  feel a burning sensation or a hot flash.

- **Peak VO2 assessment.** You'll be placed on a treadmill or a stationary
  bicycle and told to walk or pedal while inhaling and exhaling through a
  mouthpiece. This measures your body's uptake of oxygen and production of carbon dioxide.

Who gets lung transplants?

There are many diseases that damage the lungs so badly that only a transplant can help. Pulmonary hypertension is the most common diagnosis among people who receive lung transplants. In this condition blood vessels in the lung become thick and narrow, and provide a great deal of resistance to blood flow. Other common diagnoses among lung transplant patients include cystic fibrosis (an inherited disease that causes chronic lung infection and scarring), pulmonary fibrosis (scarring from tuberculosis or other lung infections), emphysema (a loss of lung elasticity that makes breathing difficult), and bronchiectasis (a chronic dilation of the bronchi—the large air tubes—which can lead to lung infection and inflammation).

Qualifying for lung and heart-lung transplants

Depending on the type of lung disease and its cause, patients may receive a single-lung transplant, a double-lung transplant, or a heart-lung transplant. James Theodore, MD, a pulmonologist and medical director of the lung transplant program at Stanford University Medical Center, explains that the transplant team has to decide whether a given patient is a candidate for lung transplant at all, and if so, what form of the surgery he or she should receive.

> *There are about a hundred different disease processes that can affect the lung. Single-lung transplants can be done for any condition providing it's not a suppurative condition, that is, where you have chronic infection in the lungs such as bronchiectasis or cystic fibrosis. We'll do single-lung transplants if you have emphysema or if you have pulmonary fibrosis, for example. But we don't transplant where the disease process is part of the multi-system disease. By multi-system I mean, say you have an individual who has lupus, and who has lung disease, brain disease, and kidney disease, as part of it. You wouldn't necessarily want to transplant that person.*

There is some controversy in the field about when to do a single-lung transplant, and when to transplant both lungs. Dr. Theodore explains that at Stanford the transplant team believes there are definite advantages to double-lung transplants:

The double-lung transplant, at least at Stanford, we prefer to do in patients with suppurative disease, and with pulmonary hypertension, although some programs will do single-lung transplants in the latter group.

I think our feeling is if you do a single-lung transplant for pulmonary hypertension, the whole blood flow or entire cardiac output will go to the transplanted lung. If something happens to the transplanted lung, then the patient is in real big trouble from the very beginning, and survival is going to be very difficult. The risks are much greater. In the long term, if one gets one of the major long-term complications such as chronic rejection—and most patients who are long-term survivors are going to get that in one form or another—then you basically don't have any reserve in the non-transplanted lung. So these people will get into trouble much sooner.

The main argument on the other side is that in double-lung transplants the donor lungs can benefit only a single recipient, while with single-lung transplants one donor can potentially benefit two lung recipients. In addition, double-lung surgery takes longer and is more complex than single-lung surgery.

Lungs can also become damaged as a result of heart failure, and conversely hearts can be damaged as a result of lung disease. When the heart and both lungs are damaged, surgeons may choose to transplant all three organs at once. This too is controversial in some quarters, Dr. Theodore points out:

Some argue against heart-lung transplants, so you can benefit three patients instead of one. You put a heart in one person, and two lungs in two others. But some people need them all.

As with heart transplants, age is an important consideration in qualifying for lung or heart-lung transplants, says Dr. Theodore:

After the age of 50 we don't like to do heart-lung transplants, because at that point, the incidence of people having multi-system disease or advanced vascular disease is much greater. Although age isn't an absolute criterion, certainly age does become an important factor.

We do single lungs in people up to age 60, although we've done them in people who are a little older as long as they're fit. Fifty-five is our upper limit for double lungs and 50 for heart-lungs. Other programs are doing them up to 65. It's based on the experience that we want to transplant the best possible candidates. The theory is that we have to have patients with end-stage disease, but we don't want desperate situations. So, you have to be sick enough to need it, but healthy enough to survive it. I'm talking about long-term survival with the full capacity for rehabilitation. If there is no chance for rehabilitation, then I don't think it's worth doing a transplant. That's our basic philosophy.

If you are denied a place on one hospital's waiting list because of your age, you may wish to investigate whether other transplant programs—either in your area or in another to which you can travel—may have more liberal criteria.

Many tests are performed to determine whether a person is a candidate for lung or heart-lung transplant. These may include:

- **Pulmonary function test (PFT).** This is really a series of tests, some of which will be performed while you are exercising, intended to determine the maximum amount of air you can inhale and exhale, the time it takes to do this, and the ability of your lungs to transmit oxygen and remove carbon dioxide from your blood. Together these tests determine the extent of your lung disease and the amount of oxygen you need to perform the normal tasks of daily living.

- **High-resolution chest CT scan.** This specialized x-ray will provide a detailed picture of the inside of your chest. It will help determine the extent of your lung disease.

- **Cardiovascular tests.** These will include most of the same tests used for heart-transplant patients. They are described in the previous section.

Heart-transplant surgery

It wasn't so many years ago—the late 1960s—that each individual heart transplant made international headlines, and the names of both the surgeon and the recipient became household words. Heart transplants long ago retreated from being on the frontiers of medical science. For skilled surgeons it isn't even an especially difficult operation to perform anymore.

While it may be comforting for heart recipients to consider that the surgery has come a long way since its beginnings, remember that it is still major surgery. In this section, we'll describe what the medical team will be doing to you just before, during, and after surgery.

When your transplant team hears that a donor heart has become available, they send a highly experienced team of surgeons and surgical nurses to retrieve it. This team will come from your hospital whether the donor is at a small community hospital or a major medical center with a transplant team of its own.

Cooperating with separate teams there to recover the other organs, your team will first clamp the blood vessels going to and from the donor heart, and then they'll pump in a cold protective solution that makes the heart stop beating. The heart is removed from the donor's body and placed into a plastic bag filled with ice and a preservative solution, and that bag is placed in an ordinary picnic cooler for transport back to your hospital.

Meanwhile you will be called to the hospital if you're not there already, and your team will take care to coordinate the timing of your surgery so that you'll be ready when the donor heart arrives. For the best outcome, the goal is to have your new heart put in your body as quickly as possible, to minimize any damage to the organ, while at the same time ensuring that you do not have to be in surgery any longer than necessary.

As transplant nurse Joan Miller explains, in many cases the recipient is prepped for surgery even before the donor heart arrives in the hospital:

> The way it's supposed to work is the recipient goes to the operating room, they start intravenous lines, and they get him ready, but they don't necessarily put him under anesthesia until the team at the donor hospital calls and says, "It's a go. The heart looks good. We're going to take it, and this is what time we think we will be back."

> The only time we would deliberately put somebody under anesthesia and start the surgery before that is if (1) we were really pretty sure that everything was going to work out, that everything we heard about the donor was positive, and (2) if the recipient had had previous open heart surgery. Those people are gong to have a lot of adhesions and scarring, and their surgery is going to take longer. Sometimes the surgeons would begin earlier on them, just so they would be ready when the donor heart got there.

Rest assured, however, that although the surgeons might start the operation, they would never take any irrevocable steps—such as removing your old heart—before the donor heart had arrived in the hospital. That's because they need to guard against the possibility that the donor team could be involved in a car accident (for example) while delivering the heart.

Once you're fully anesthetized, the skin on your upper chest will be shaved, and the area will be disinfected with an iodine scrub. Other parts of your body away from your chest will be draped with sterile cloths. The surgeon will make an incision to expose your breastbone and will saw through the middle of the breastbone. This allows him to pull your ribs out of the way and expose your heart.

The next step is to attach you to a heart-lung machine, which will take over the job of adding oxygen to, removing carbon dioxide from, and circulating your blood until the new heart is fully inserted. After injecting you with anticoagulants to prevent your blood from clotting in the heart-lung machine, the surgeon will attach two tubes to the right side of your heart to collect unoxygenated blood, and two others to your aorta to return oxygenated blood.

The heart-lung machine is also used to warm or cool your blood and therefore your body. Once the machine has taken over your circulation, your body temperature will be cooled to 78° F, a chilly 20 degrees below normal. This prevents damage to other organs during the surgery.

The surgeons then remove your heart. The donor heart is removed from its bag, and surgeons begin the delicate task of connecting the donor heart's blood vessels to your own. A great deal of surgical skill is involved in this procedure. Surgeons call the connection between two vessels an anastomosis (the plural is anastomoses), and making a good, tight anastomosis is one of the highest expressions of the surgeon's art. Surgeons take enormous care to match up the vessels and to suture them together tightly, so there are no leaks. Often they're required to sculpt the donor vessels and the recipient's, so that they match up well

The surgeons ascertain that there are no air bubbles in the new heart and they make the final connections. After that, the new heart often starts contracting all by itself. Sometimes, though, the new heart takes a while to recover, and occasionally the surgeons have to shock the heart to get it going. While this is happening, the surgeons use the heart-lung machine to warm your blood to normal body temperature.

Your new heart will not have normal connections to your nervous system, since those will have been severed when the old heart was removed.

Unfortunately, these nerve connections cannot be reattached. One possible short-term consequence of this is that your new heart may not be beating fast enough. If this is the case, the surgeons may administer medications to increase your heart rate, and they may also insert a temporary pacemaker to help your heart keep its beat. The pacemaker is normally removed within several days. (We'll discuss the surprisingly minor long-term consequences of the severed nerve connections later in this chapter.)

Once your heart is beating well, you'll be gradually weaned from the heart-lung machine. Its connections are removed, and then the surgeons begin closing up your wounds. Drainage tubes are inserted in your chest (to be removed within a few days.) The severed halves of your breastbone are wired together, and the skin and overlying tissue are sewn up using special thread that will dissolve on its own after the wound has healed.

When the operation is over, you're wheeled into the recovery room, still deeply anesthetized. You're placed on a ventilator, a machine that pushes air into and out of your lungs through a tube in your throat. You'll feel that tube as you gradually regain consciousness over the next several hours. Most patients find the ventilator and the breathing tube uncomfortable, and they also prevent you from speaking. You'll do better if you can relax and avoid fighting against the action of the ventilator. Fortunately, the medical team is almost always able to wean you from the ventilator within 24 hours, allowing you to speak and to breathe on your own.

Lung and heart-lung transplant surgery

Lung transplantation became available more recently than heart transplants, with the first successful transplants taking place in the early 1980s. Lung transplants are less common than heart transplants. In 1998, surgeons in the US performed 849 lung transplants and 45 heart-lung transplants.

As with heart transplants, in lung transplants there must be careful coordination between donor and recipient surgical teams. One thing that potential recipients need to know is that healthy donor lungs are more rare than are hearts. That's because lungs are more likely than hearts to get damaged in accidents. Even small bruises or punctures will render a potential donor lung unsuitable.

The surgical details are similar to those of heart transplants, described in the previous section. Sometimes, just as in heart transplants, lung transplant recipients will be placed on a heart-lung machine during surgery. Other times, the remaining diseased lung will be breathing for you while the new lung is being attached.

If you are receiving a single lung, the surgeon must make an anastomosis or connection between the cut ends of the bronchus. He must also make connections between the cut ends of the pulmonary artery and the pulmonary veins.

If you're receiving two lungs, the surgeon will make two sets of anastomoses for the pulmonary arteries and veins. Regarding the airway connection, the surgeon has two choices. He can either transplant each lung separately, creating two anastomoses, one for each of the bronchi, or he can transplant both lungs as a unit, still attached with the windpipe (the trachea), and create a single anastomosis at the trachea.

Dr. Theodore explains that the latter technique is rarely used these days:

> The way that it's done now is that you do one side and then the other side, so you basically do two single-lung transplants in sequence. In the past, surgeons would transplant both lungs at the same time with a tracheal anastomosis. But there are more complications at the anastomotic sites with that operation, so hardly anyone does it anymore.

In heart-lung transplants, the heart and both lungs are removed from the donor as a single unit—a so-called heart-lung block. In the early days of this surgery all three organs were inserted as a single block into the recipient, but that technique is rarely used today. Instead, the two lungs and the heart are separated and are inserted one by one.

Surgeons also used to perform "domino" surgery. In domino surgery the recipient would have diseased lungs but a healthy heart. The healthy heart and diseased lungs would be removed and replaced by the donor's heart-lung block. Since there was no point in wasting a perfectly good heart, that heart would be transplanted to another recipient. Domino surgery is virtually never performed these days, since surgeons have found more effective ways of performing single-lung and double-lung transplants.

Although it's still experimental, some lung transplant teams have been successful in performing living-donor lung transplants for certain patients.

Recipients are typically people who need double-lung transplants, and each recipient requires two donors. One person donates the left lung's lower lobe, and the other donates the right lung's lower lobe. For more information, see Chapter 13, *Living Donors*.

Immediately after surgery

Heart transplant surgery typically takes about four to five hours. Lung transplant surgery can take longer—five to ten hours is not unusual, especially if it's a double-lung or heart-lung transplant. If you're the patient, you won't be aware of the time passing, but your family certainly will. They'll most likely be waiting in a special area near the operating room.

Families need to be prepared for a long wait and the likely appearance of the patient when they first get to see him. Joan Miller explains that the family will be given a progress report as soon as the surgery is completed, if not before:

> The family stays in the waiting rooms outside the operating room. If it's a long case, someone may come out and give them some sort of bulletin halfway through, otherwise they just wait until the surgery's done. And then the surgeons come out and talk to them, let them know how it went, how their family member is doing, and it's usually another 30 to 45 minutes after that before the patient comes out.

> Once the patient's in the intensive care unit and settled, the staff will let the family come in and see him. That's usually a quick visit and it's usually traumatic for the family because patients are quite pale and cold from being cooled during the surgery. There are all sorts of lines going into and out of the patient, the ventilator is still going, and it can be frightening.

As a transplant coordinator, Joan Miller has seen many patients after heart-transplant surgery. She describes what happens as the anesthesia wears off:

> The patient wakes up quickly after surgery. Depending on how they respond to anesthesia, it could be a little longer for some people, but usually they're awake pretty quickly. If they get back from the operating room at 7 in the morning, for example, they're often up in a chair by early afternoon. Few of them remember much of anything about that day. But they can almost always respond appropriately, and they recognize their family.

Family members may find that post-surgical amnesia to be quite disconcerting. A patient's wife may have a pleasant conversation with him that first day in which she tells him he had the transplant and came out of the surgery fine. From his responses, it will be quite clear that he understands everything that was said. But the next morning, the first question out of his mouth may be, "Did I have the transplant?" This may seem worrisome, but it's actually quite normal.

While patients will normally experience some pain following heart or lung transplant surgery, in most cases this pain is surprisingly manageable, notes Ms. Miller:

> Patients are actually not in a great deal of pain after the surgery. There's still some residual anesthesia, and having the sternum cut is not as painful as having the abdomen cut because the muscles are different. When you consider what was done, they really request and are given a very moderate amount of pain medicine. They'll get a little bit of Demerol [a narcotic pain reliever] or something intravenously, and then as soon as they're on oral medicines they'll switch to something for pain that they can take by mouth.

Your doctors will be watching you very closely for the first two or three days after surgery. Stanford University cardiologist Sharon A. Hunt, MD, explains:

> It's really a very complex period of time that takes a lot of clinical attention and insight. You're looking for the patient to stay well, to maintain blood pressure, to make urine.

> It varies, but they're in the intensive care unit (ICU) two to three to four days. Then they're in the hospital another few days up to a week or so.

During recovery in the hospital the patient will be placed on immunosuppressive (anti-rejection) medications, some at very high doses. Some transplant teams even start one or two of these medications pre-operatively. Here Dr. Hunt describes a typical immunosuppressive regimen (for more detail on the drugs she mentions, see Chapter 8, Anti-Rejection Drugs):

> It often involves the use of "induction" therapy with a monoclonal antibody called OKT3. Then there's the variable introduction of cyclosporine, preoperative starting of azathioprine, and the use of steroids, initially in low doses, and a bump up in dose after the OKT3 is done. Management is incredibly individual. Some patients come into the transplant

a lot sicker than others and demand a lot of micro-management, and some walk in and do fine with standard therapy.

These anti-rejection drugs make people highly susceptible to infection. At some transplant centers, visitors are told to wear surgical caps, gowns, face masks, and even booties while in the patient's room. However, Ms. Miller remarks that at Stanford these precautions are seen as overkill:

> *We no longer require that visitors wear surgical gowns. The nurses in the cardiac ICU did a study a few years ago, and there was no difference in infection rate between gowning and not gowning. So we practice universal precautions—such as hand washing before contact with any patient—and that's it. We don't even use face masks unless somebody is infected or thinks they have a cold. But when the patients leave the room they have to wear masks because we never know whom they might run into.*

Recovery

Transplant recipients vary in the amount of time they spend in the intensive care unit and then in a regular hospital room before being released to go home. Joan Miller explains what happens if everything goes well:

> *What we would refer to as a straightforward heart patient—somebody who followed the plan and had no complications would probably be out of the ICU in 36 hours, 48 at the most, out on what we call the step-down unit for three to five days, and home on the sixth or seventh day after surgery.*

Double-lung recipient Kathryn M. Flynn was unable to breathe without the ventilator, so she spent a longer time in the hospital:

> *I had a hard time getting off the ventilator, so I was in the ICU about eleven days. That's a lot longer than average for a lung transplant. Most people are out in 24 hours now. Every time they tried to take out the line, I couldn't breathe on my own, and so they'd have to put it back in. They tried BiPAP [bilateral positive air pressure] too, and I was on that for a while. BiPAP is some kind of weird breathing device where they shoot oxygen at you at a high speed. After eleven days, it finally worked, and I was able to get off the vent.*

> Altogether I was in the hospital two-and-a-half weeks. I didn't feel better right away. I was pretty weak from being in the ICU for that long. But once I went home and got into rehab, it only took about a week until I felt better.

One thing most transplant recipients can be certain of is that their nurses will be hard taskmasters almost as soon as the anesthesia wears off. As Ms. Miller explains:

> We like to get them up and walking around pretty quickly. There's a chance they might take a few steps late that night, but certainly by the next morning they'd be walking around the bed, or they'd be up and moving. It's the best thing physiologically for the body to get up and standing upright. It's also the leading preventive measure to stop the formation of blood clots, and it helps you breathe better. Everything works better when they're standing upright. It gets their stomachs working so they're ready to eat a little quicker, and the faster you can get them up and going the better off they are. Psychologically, it's an incredible boost to patients and their families.
>
> They're usually not able to use the bathroom by themselves at first. They come back with a catheter in because they're pretty sleepy and groggy, but that usually comes out that first day. Regarding bowel movements, it could be a couple days before the gut's working regularly. In ICU they probably use a bedside commode because of getting through all the equipment to the bathroom. But the minute they're out on the step-down unit, they're walking to the bathroom.

Dr. Theodore says that he sees the best results in patients who are highly motivated and push themselves to get well:

> It depends on the individual, but lung-transplant patients tend to feel pretty good, fairly early. Highly motivated people who can deal with a lot of pain can push themselves, and if there are no problems, they come around pretty quickly. With others who have a problem with pain, then you have to find yourself using excessive amounts of pain medication. They're not motivated, they don't push themselves very hard. We try to get our patients mobilized and exercising and walking very, very, very early. We don't like them lying around.

Here, Jim Gleason describes the exercise regimen he and his fellow heart-transplant patients followed after their surgeries:

> As soon as we came out of the sleep after surgery, actually the next day, nurses helped us sit up and start with the exercise of slight movement—talk about starting all over—and we thought we had been in decent condition. Within days we were walking the course again. But we now had a time frame for our goal—ten days if all went well, and we could go home.
>
> That's all we had to hear. After all these weeks, the thought of going home was a real incentive. When we found out that one of the conditions for going home after surgery was the passing of a test to show we could get around, including going up some stairs, the pattern of our walking rounds was modified to include the climbing up/down of stairs at the end of the unit.
>
> The steroids that prevented heart rejection also played havoc with the body muscles, especially those in the legs. These muscles would turn to Jell-O almost overnight if we skipped our routine, and then you had to start over, rebuilding that Jell-O into supporting leg muscles again. Ouch!

Once you have left the ICU, members of the transplant team will come around frequently to teach you and your primary caregiver all the things you need to know about living with a transplant. Joan Miller describes how these sessions are conducted:

> When they've left the ICU and are in the step-down unit, that's the point where my group and I step in. We start coming around and introducing ourselves. We have some printed information that we give to the patients and their families. Usually the first day or so we give it to the family member so the patient doesn't have to keep track of it. It gives the family some information to read during a lot of the down time they have.
>
> They get two books. One's a small book for the patient to have at the bedside to help them learn their medicine. The minute they wake up and are taking medicines by mouth, the nurses at the bedside go over every medicine with them as they take it: "This is your cyclosporine, this is what it does, these are the side effects." And they have a little book they can refer to and they can make notes. They're supposed to open the book, watch the nurse, and get involved.

They also have a bigger book of about 50 pages, the Patient Teaching Manual. That's the one the family usually keeps. It covers a great deal of information about transplants: post-op rejection, infection, diet, exercise, outpatient clinic, wellness, coming to clinic, annual studies, and a huge section on drug interactions. It's very informative, and it's our primary teaching tool.

Often we'll just sit with them for an hour or so, every other day, and ask, "What questions do you have? How are things going? What do you not understand? Do you have a place to live? Are you all settled?" We also ask, "Where do you get your prescriptions filled?" so we can start making plans to have all their medicines ready for them when they head out the door.

While most hospital patients are simply handed their medications by the nurse at the appropriate time, transplant patients are given far more responsibility. The thinking is that since you're going to have to be responsible for taking a large number of pills every day for the rest of your life once you get home, there's no time like the present for getting used to this. Lisa G. Levin, a nurse coordinator at Stanford University's cardiothoracic surgery department explains:

From the time they start taking oral medications, we ask them to give themselves their own medication. They have a tremendous number of drugs that they have to take once they leave the hospital, and if they can't demonstrate that they can safely administer them, then we can't discharge them. We need to have the bedside nurses who work with them 24 hours a day verify the patients are delivering their drugs appropriately. And if they're not then we have to find family members who can step in to help them.

Team members will also tell you what symptoms to keep an eye on. Joan Miller says that people tend to focus on avoiding rejection when it would probably be more productive to focus on avoiding infection.

Almost all patients and their families want to focus on rejection and how to prevent it and how to spot it early. Unfortunately, it's really hard for patients to know when they're in rejection. Rejection has almost no symptoms in adults. We try and focus their attention on infection because that's the leading cause of death and morbidity. A patient is often the very first person to know if she's getting an infection. She'll know if she has a *fever, a cough, burning when she urinates, etc., little signs that could tell her she's becoming infected.*

Dr. Hunt agrees:

> *We ask patients to be very alert for signs of infection, and we ask them to monitor their home blood pressure since most of them get high blood pressure afterwards. And if there's any tendency to high blood sugars, we'll often ask them to monitor blood sugars at home.*
>
> *Generally we have them come back twice a week for clinics, and taper back to once a week after a few weeks if they're okay. They get three surveillance biopsies within the first month, then they go down to every other week for about another month, then monthly for the first six months.*

Lung recipients will have a similar post-transplant regimen, says Dr. Theodore:

> *We do the first surveillance biopsy within two weeks after the transplant. We monitor their lung function very closely. We monitor their blood gases. You're going to see changes in lung function and blood gases at some point, and it could indicate there may be something going on, but that's more reliable the further out you are from the surgery because then you're past a lot of the acute changes associated with the surgery.*
>
> *After they're discharged, we see patients twice a week for about the first three weeks, and then we go to once a week, then once every two weeks. We keep them near the hospital for about 90 days. We have to do surveillance bronchoscopies to check for lung rejection, and if they've had a heart-lung transplant, then you have to monitor their heart, and you'll need heart biopsies to watch for heart rejection. You have to monitor their livers, their kidneys, because of all the complications that are associated with the drugs that they take. The risk of infection is always great. Lungs are exposed to the atmosphere, so they run a greater risk of getting infection than other organs, so you have to pay a little closer attention to things like aspergillus, pneumocystis, and various kinds of fungal infections.*

Both lung and heart recipients also need to learn how to deal with the fact that their new organs don't have intact nerve connections to the rest of the body. In the case of the heart, it's these nerve connections that cause the heart to speed up when we're excited or when we exercise. In response to excitement, our adrenal glands release hormones like adrenaline, which also increase heart rate, but this takes a bit longer than a nerve connection. It's advisable to warm up slowly when you're exercising—and even to avoid standing up rapidly—to let your heart catch up with your activity.

Jim Gleason explains that it was fairly easy for him to get used to this:

> *The most interesting side effect was an adjustment to the lack of nerve connections between the new heart and this body. In this case, the transplant team's education was right on, and it was fairly easy to adjust to the regimen of standing up, then waiting until blood was moving to the brain, before walking. Any time this was forgotten, the body sent signals in the form of dizziness (lightheadedness) to remind me. A slight wait, and all was ready to go again. It was forecasted that this would last for years, if not my whole life. My experience was that by month three, some-how the body had found alternate paths of communications and it was no longer a problem.*

In the case of lung recipients, the missing nerve connections are the ones that encourage us to cough after we've inhaled irritants. You will need to remind yourself to cough at regular intervals, so these irritants can be expelled. Failure to do so can result in an increased risk of lung infection. The missing nerve connections also are partly responsible for increasing breathing rate during exercise. At first you'll have to learn to consciously increase your breathing rate during exercise. Within three to six months, for unknown reasons, the body seems to find alternate ways of handling this without conscious intervention.

Heart and lung transplant recipients have a good chance of living full lives. According to study conducted by the United Network for Organ Sharing (UNOS) of patients transplanted between October 1987 and December 1997, of 21,776 heart recipients, 83.5 percent survived at least one year and 72.1 percent survived at least four years. Of 5,277 lung recipients, 73.9 percent survived one year and 49.5 percent survived four years. Of 600 heart-lung recipients, 64.6 percent survived one year and 45.8 percent survived four years.

Your mileage may vary, as they say, but survival rates are going nowhere but up. (One thing to remember about these numbers is that they simply give the total percentage of survivors at given intervals, and are not corrected for cause of death. Some people die for reasons having nothing to do with their transplants.) You'll find much more information about increasing your chances of survival in Chapter 9, *Living with a Transplant*.

The statistics clearly don't tell the whole story. If there's one thing that's apparent, it's that heart and lung transplants change people's lives. Joan Miller has seen it all:

> We've run the gamut from people hardly waking up, to people who wake up saying, "God is in my life! It's a miracle. I'm going to do good works!" It's really sweet to watch. They come down off their high eventually and resume their normal lives. The lung patients will look at their fingernails, and say, "Oh, my gracious. They're not blue anymore!" The heart patients can feel the circulation coming back out to their fingers and toes and their brain. It's amazing how good they feel and how quickly. Even though they're still pretty sick and they've got a lot of recovering and rehabilitation to do, they really feel better almost immediately.

CHAPTER 5

Liver Transplants

THIS CHAPTER DISCUSSES WHAT SORT OF PEOPLE will be considered for liver transplants, and it describes what happens before, during, and after surgery.

While the chapter focuses on issues specific to liver recipients, it contains information of interest to the recipients of other transplants as well. Likewise, liver recipients may find relevant material in Chapters 4 and 6, which focus on heart, lung, kidney, and pancreas transplants. Although the details of the transplant surgeries themselves are obviously different, all transplant patients, no matter what organ they receive, share a good many common experiences. This is particularly true of post-surgical experiences, and you will want to peruse those sections of all three chapters.

It's important to realize that different transplant teams have different ways of doing things. Depending on where you have your transplant done, some of the details presented in the following pages may vary.

If you're interested in liver transplants, *The Wall Street Journal* reporter Scott McCartney has written a wonderful book, *Defying the Gods: Inside the New Frontiers of Organ Transplants*. It chronicles the history of the procedure, discusses its ethics and economics, and tells the exciting, inspirational, and occasionally heartbreaking stories of four people awaiting transplants. Although McCartney's book is a bit out of date—liver transplants have become more routine in the years since it was published—it is still well worth a look.

Who gets liver transplants?

The most common reason for liver transplants in adults is some form of cirrhosis. Cirrhosis is a progressive scarring of the liver, often accompanied by the formation of fatty deposits. Cirrhosis has several different causes, including alcoholism, drug abuse, and viral diseases such as hepatitis B and hepatitis C. Transplants may also be required when the liver is damaged by the ingestion of certain toxins, such as those found in the deathcap mushroom, *Amanita phalloides*. Cancer can also damage the liver badly enough to require transplant, but as we will see in the next section, many cancer patients are excluded from transplantation.

Biliary atresia—a congenital blockage of the bile ducts—is the most common reason for liver transplantation in children.

One of the main functions of the liver is the production of bile, a thick, yellow fluid that helps in the digestion of fats in the intestines. Accumulation of bile is often one of the first symptoms of liver disease, as it results in jaundice—a yellowing of the skin, the whites of the eyes, and the mucous membranes.

The liver removes toxins from the blood and also produces thousands of enzymes that are secreted into the bloodstream to be circulated throughout the body. The lack of those enzymes can cause many problems in people with liver disease. For example, it's the liver that produces the factors responsible for clotting the blood. Without those clotting factors, even a small scratch can bleed uncontrollably.

Other common symptoms of liver disease include an accumulation of fluid in the abdomen that's called ascites (pronounced a-SIGH-tees), extremely itchy skin, a lack of appetite, disruptions in sleep patterns, and in advanced stages, serious cognitive impairment.

Suzan Best was only in her early 30s when she discovered that a hepatitis C infection was destroying her liver:

> I was in and out of the hospital for two years or so. I knew it was getting worse, but I didn't understand what was really happening. I was told about what a slow death having liver failure is. I was scared. I had ascites really, really bad, so I looked like I was nine months pregnant for a very long time. It wouldn't go away. I was very rarely able to walk around. The last year I had to have help. I was bedridden. I couldn't eat, and when I did eat I had to force myself, and even then it would be maybe half a sandwich. I felt like I was doomed. I felt, "Why me? I'm only thirty-three years old." Toward the end I was giving up, but I still had hope. They never really told me outright how long I had to live. But I found out later that they told my husband I had two to six months if I didn't get a transplant.

In 1998, 4,450 people received liver transplants in the US, a number that was increased significantly by living donation and by the practice of splitting donated livers so that two recipients can benefit from a single liver.

Qualifying for a liver transplant

Not everyone with liver disease is a candidate for a liver transplant. If you're referred as a potential candidate for transplant, the transplant team will conduct a number of medical tests to ensure that you need a liver and that you'll be likely to survive the operation. Although some of the qualifying criteria can seem harsh in individual cases, transplant teams focus on what will work. They want to maximize the results from a precious and scarce resource—donated organs—and make sure that a life will be saved.

One thing to remember is that not all transplant teams use the same criteria. If one medical center decides that you are not a candidate for transplant, you may want to investigate whether you might have access to other medical centers that use a somewhat different set of standards.

When you're referred for a transplant evaluation, you'll be sent for many tests, and you'll have appointments with several different physicians, says Rae Ann Hopkins Berry, LCSW, a social worker at Stanford University:

> During the initial evaluation, the patient has a lot of medical tests.
> He sees a hepatologist (a liver specialist), a surgeon, and often he sees a
> cardiologist. We need to know about more than just the liver because
> we're going to immune-suppress the person. Suppose there's a tiny tumor
> somewhere else in the body that normally would be causing no problem at
> all. But when a person is immune-suppressed, it could just grow like wild-
> fire and be fatal. We also look for other diseases that might be affected
> when the patient is immune-suppressed.

If the tests detect cancer outside of the patient's liver, he will most likely not be a candidate for transplant. But the situation may be different if the cancer is confined to the liver, says Emmet B. Keeffe, MD, Medical Director of the Liver Transplant Program at Stanford University Medical Center:

> One area that has been challenging is patients who have cirrhosis
> complicated by liver cancer—hepatoma or hepatocellular carcinoma.
> Those patients need to be transplanted in a timely fashion so that they
> can have the liver removed before the tumor spreads beyond the liver.

Because of the long waiting time for transplants today, that's a particular challenge, although we try to slow down the growth of the tumor by using chemoembolization. That's a radiologic procedure where the radiologist puts a catheter through the groin up to the liver and injects chemotherapy together with a material that makes the chemotherapy stay in the area of the tumor for a period of time.

There are several other medical conditions that can exclude someone from transplant, says Dr. Keeffe, but some conditions that used to be exclusionary no longer are:

Other considerations that might tend to exclude somebody often relate to what we call co-morbidities—other simultaneous medical conditions. Let's say, for example, somebody has had a heart attack in the past, but the heart attack has been treated. We have to do a careful assessment in this case regarding the cause of their heart disease and the prognosis for their heart disease. So we have to do our best to understand the medical problem and understand whether or not that will interfere with success after transplantation.

Years ago, when the results were poor for liver transplantation, some transplant centers excluded patients with chronic hepatitis B. Our old program had never done that because we were always optimistic we could achieve good results using the strategy of administering hepatitis B immune globulin. Now transplantation with hepatitis B is no longer controversial. The outcome is quite good.

Patients who are alcoholics or drug abusers and are actively drinking or using drugs will also be excluded from consideration for transplant. But someone who can demonstrate a certain time period of sobriety and participation in rehabilitation may be listed, if a psychiatrist or alcoholism expert decides that the patient is recovering from his previous addiction. Many programs require six months of sobriety, but in other programs the time period may be longer, shorter, or variable depending on the individual patient. Some programs require participation in alcohol rehabilitation for all alcoholics, but in others that requirement can be waived at the discretion of a rehabilitation expert. (See Chapter 2, *The System*, for more on this.)

Dr. Keeffe emphasizes that there are good medical reasons for the requirement for sobriety:

This is a medical decision. If a patient is continuing to abuse alcohol, that means they're going to be intoxicated, and it's likely they're not going to take their medicines, their liver will undergo rejection, and they will damage the graft that they received. We want patients to be sober and compliant so that they're going to take appropriate care of their new liver in terms of follow-up visits, regular use of medication, and so on.

We verify that they're not drinking by random alcohol screens using urine or blood tests. In our own particular program, we have patients sign a contract in which they agree to go to their local laboratory within four hours of a phone call for a random alcohol check to confirm compliance.

Psychiatrist Kathy L. Coffman, MD, of St. Vincent Medical Center in Los Angeles, points out that active alcoholism won't necessarily disqualify someone forever, as long as he takes steps to get sober and stay that way:

Some programs will just turn them down flat if they're still using, and that's the end of it. But many of the programs will try to salvage those patients by getting them involved in a treatment program and evaluating them later down the line after they have been clean and sober for a period of time. In our program we try to get patients involved in rehabilitation early on in the process.

Age is another factor that may tend to disqualify someone from a liver transplant, although this is less of a problem now than in the past, explains Dr. Keeffe:

It used to be, in the early, early days, the cut-off was age 45, and then age 50, and then age 60, and now it's somewhere between age 60 and 70. However, we pay attention to the physiologic age rather than the chronologic age of the patient. The concept is that there is a limited supply of organs and we wouldn't want to use up an organ if someone is only going to live another three to five years.

Rae Ann Berry explains the evaluation conference that's held after all the tests are complete:

When everything is completed and we have all the paperwork—and this usually takes several weeks at least—we have a meeting of the liver transplant team. We go over patients who have recently been seen, and we make a decision about whether the person is a candidate for transplant or not. We can accept candidates or we can turn them down, which *we don't like to do. There has to be a reason. Sometimes we defer a patient so a problem can be worked on, after which he can become a candidate. After becoming a candidate, he is put on the list to wait his turn for a donor liver, and sometimes that wait is up to four years or more. In northern California, the lists are very long.*

Liver transplant surgery

Although liver transplant surgery is becoming increasingly common, it is still one of the most complex and demanding operations that a surgeon can perform.

Most transplanted livers come from cadaveric donors, although an increasing number—especially for children—come from living donors. Of the 4,450 liver transplants performed in the US in 1998, there were 4,384 cadaveric and 66 living donor liver transplants. As described more fully in Chapter 13, *Living Donors*, surgeons are able to safely take a part of one person's liver and implant it into another. Since healthy livers regenerate easily, the remaining part of the donor's liver will grow to its former size, and the small piece transplanted into a child will grow as the child grows.

Living donor liver transplants grew out of the practice of splitting cadaveric livers. Dr. Keeffe explains when and why this is done:

> *Split livers are being done with an increasing frequency now. It's a way we can really get two for one. We can retrieve an organ at Stanford and have part of the liver go to a patient at Stanford, another part go to a patient at UC San Francisco, for example, or UCLA. It's a way to help alleviate the organ shortage. Not every liver can be split. You have to give the larger portion to an adult and the smaller portion to a child. If you have a large recipient, they may need the entire liver.*

Transplant surgeon Michael Wachs, MD, of the University of Colorado Health Science Center explains that it's unlikely that both parts of a split liver will go to adult recipients:

> *The use of split liver transplants for two adults has not really taken off, because it's more difficult to split a liver directly in half into right and left sides, and figure out all the complexities of the anatomy to make both sides work.*

When your transplant team hears that a donor liver has become available, they will send a highly experienced team of surgeons and surgical nurses to retrieve it. This team will come from your hospital whether the donor is at a small community hospital or a major medical center with a transplant team of its own.

Cooperating with other teams there to procure other organs, your team will remove the liver and place it in a plastic bag filled with a special preservative solution. For transport they'll place that bag in an ordinary picnic cooler filled with ice, and they'll return to your hospital.

It used to be that livers could survive for only six hours without circulating blood, so transplants had to be performed quickly, and donor organs had to be procured fairly close to the recipient. But as Dr. Keeffe explains, a new preservative solution is increasing the time that a liver can be outside the body, which means that nowadays livers can be transported practically anywhere in the US for transplant:

> There's a new organ preservation solution called the Wisconsin Solution. That solution now allows longer preservation, even up to as long as twelve or eighteen hours. But the longer a liver is preserved, the less of a chance it will function as well. We still like to get transplants done in less than twelve hours if possible.

While the donor team is out retrieving the liver, you'll be admitted to the hospital. You should know that it's actually fairly common that the donor team will discover that the donor liver is not suitable for transplant. If the liver turns out to be unacceptable, you'll be discharged without receiving a transplant. But the team will want to have you in the hospital while they're making that determination to decrease the amount of time the liver will spend without a blood supply.

If the donor liver is acceptable, you'll be prepped for surgery as the transplant team awaits the arrival of the donor organ. You'll be anesthetized, and your chest will be shaved and washed with a disinfecting iodine solution. For the best outcome, the goal is to have your new liver put into your body as quickly as possible, to minimize any damage to the organ, while at the same time ensuring that you do not have to be in surgery any longer than necessary.

The liver is a large organ, and the surgeons will need to make a large incision to remove the old organ and to insert the new one. The incision will cross almost the entire width of your abdomen, just below your ribs. Once the surgeons have opened your abdominal cavity, a member of the surgical team will be delegated to pull your ribs up and out of the way with retractors, and then the surgeons can remove your old liver.

Since removing the liver involves interrupting the circulation in a large area of your body, you may be attached to a pump similar to the heart-lung machine described in Chapter 4. This pump helps create an alternate route for blood to travel from the lower body and intestines to the heart.

Removing the liver involves severing four major blood vessels and the bile duct, which carries bile from the liver to the intestines. Attaching the new liver involves creating anastomoses (connections) between the cut ends of each of those blood vessels, and surgeons must also connect the new liver's bile duct to your intestines. Creating an anastomosis is challenging for surgeons under the best of circumstances, but it's even more difficult in liver transplants because the major blood vessels are all on the bottom side of the organ, forcing surgeons to do most of their work underneath the liver.

Liver transplants can take eight to ten hours, or even longer if there are complications. The liver is easily bruised or torn, and surgeons have to watch out for this during the transplant. As previously mentioned, people with advanced liver disease often lack important blood-clotting factors, which means that liver transplant surgery can be particularly bloody. While the surgery is now much improved, in the early days of liver transplants, it was not unusual for a single operation to significantly deplete an entire city's blood supply. As surgeons have grown more skilled, this has become less of a problem. One solution is to use a special device called a CellSaver to collect blood spilled into the patient's abdomen and return it to the circulatory system.

Such techniques have been remarkably successful. In fact, in May 1999, surgeons in Belgium reported that by making several significant modifications in the surgical procedure they were able to perform a liver transplant without having to transfuse a single unit of blood. The patient was a member of the Jehovah's Witnesses, a religion that prohibits the use of any foreign blood products. The surgeons cautioned, however, that liver transplant surgery without the use of blood products will remain the exception rather than the rule.

Some liver transplant operations are still very bloody even today, and when they get bloody they take longer, as surgeons have to be painstaking in searching for, finding, and sealing off all sources of bleeding in the liver. That's what happened during Suzan Best's surgery:

> We got there around three in the morning, and they brought me into the surgery room around nine o'clock to prepare me. I was in surgery for sixteen hours. I had bleeding. I had to have more than 50 units of blood.

To reiterate, Suzan's experience was unusual. It's rare for a liver transplant to require that much blood.

Once the bleeding is under control and the anastomoses have all been made and checked, the surgeons will close your wound. Lower layers of muscle and skin will be sewn with a special suture material that dissolves as you heal. For the outermost layer, though, the surgeons will most likely use surgical staples, which look just like regular staples. While you may find it disconcerting to see a line of silver staples on your chest, long experience has proven them to be a safe and efficient alternative to sutures. And when it comes time to remove the staples, the procedure is simple, quick, and painless.

At the completion of the surgery, you'll be wheeled to the intensive care unit (ICU).

Recovery

It's in the ICU that your family will finally be able to see you. In Suzan's case, her husband John had been sitting in a waiting room with mounting anxiety for the full sixteen hours her surgery took. Members of the surgical team would occasionally fill him in on the progress of the surgery, and he became increasingly concerned as they told him about the complications they were encountering. It was an enormous relief to John when he was finally allowed to see her after surgery.

> In the ICU after surgery, she had a remarkable nurse. The ICU had one policy I disagree with. Every hour on the hour you could see your loved one for ten minutes and that's it. Well, this nurse let me see Suzan as long as I wished as long as she was on duty. The other nurse didn't like it. Even though Suzan was still in a drugged, comatose state, I just talked to her. I rubbed her head. I just wanted to make sure I was the first one that she saw when she first opened up her eyes. I wanted her to know that somebody was there.

Suzan remembers what it felt like to gradually awaken with a tube down her throat and a ventilator breathing for her:

> I wasn't in pain when I woke up. I think my first reaction was, "Where am I?" and then I realized I had a tube in my mouth, and I couldn't move. Things started clicking that I had the surgery and it's over. I remember thinking that they told me I'm going to feel the tube in my mouth, and it's going to be strange because I'm not breathing for myself. So I kind of remembered that, and I didn't freak out like they said some people do. My husband was there and my parents. It was really good to see them.

During recovery it's important for the patient to relax and let the body heal. You may experience some pain and discomfort, but that pain is treatable. Let your nurses know when you're hurting so they can give you the appropriate medications. Family members, for their part, need to be aware that in many cases what seems to be terrible misery on the part of the patient is not what it appears. Patients are often only vaguely aware of pain and discomfort during the first days after surgery.

In the early days of liver transplantation, patients could be expected to remain for extended stays in the hospital, but these days hospital stays are much shorter, says Rae Ann Berry:

> Back in 1988, we kept patients in the hospital a month whether they needed to be there or not. Now we've had some patients who've gotten out in four days, and most get out in six or seven.

Dr. Keeffe explains what happens during the week following surgery:

> Liver transplant patients now average one to two days in the ICU. Hospitalization averages, in our own program, seven to eight days. Then they stay in the nearby area for another two to four weeks for a careful follow-up and adjustment of medication. Then, maybe six weeks or so after transplant, they are usually discharged back to wherever they come from.
>
> Their time in the hospital is spent recovering in terms of the wounds and the surgery, and allowing the new liver to begin to function. We also begin to adjust the immunosuppressive medications. Then, as an outpatient, it's further adjustment of the immunosuppressive medications, making sure the wound heals properly without infection, and undergoing

rehabilitation and beginning to gain strength back if the patient has been
severely weakened by the liver disease.

Suzan Best recalls that despite the rigors of surgery, she started feeling relief from her liver disease immediately:

> *I felt much, much better, even while I was in the hospital in the week*
> *after the surgery. As far as pain, most of the time it was dulled pain. They*
> *didn't give me big strong pain killers. The incision was painful. If I turned*
> *a certain way it pulled the staples, and that would hurt. I felt weak more*
> *than anything. But every day I became stronger. I had an appetite like*
> *you wouldn't believe. I could actually eat, and I enjoyed it. I felt mentally*
> *better because I didn't have the feelings I had before, and my skin didn't*
> *itch like it did. I could think straight.*
>
> *I was up and walking probably the third or fourth day. They had a*
> *physical therapist come in and help me. My husband was there all the*
> *time. He stayed in the room, and he helped me get up if I needed help,*
> *which I did at first, but I was never forced to do anything. I wanted to get*
> *up, and if I needed help I'd ask for it. I think that's what helped me—*
> *instead of just laying in bed, I wanted to get up.*
>
> *One month later, I still have a big appetite. I eat three meals a day*
> *plus in between.*

During your recovery, the doctors will monitor you closely. They'll be watching your blood tests for evidence that the new liver is functioning normally and producing bile. They'll be giving you high doses of immunosuppressive medications at first, but they'll start reducing the doses almost immediately.

Other members of the transplant team will be instructing you on living with your transplant. They'll teach you about your medications, and you'll assume responsibility for taking them. You'll be up and walking around quickly, and you're likely to be amazed at how fast your strength returns.

Liver transplant patients have an excellent record of living full lives. According to a study conducted by the United Network for Organ Sharing (UNOS) of patients transplanted between October 1987 and December 1997, of 32,192 liver recipients, 81.8 percent survived at least one year and 73.3 percent survived at least four years. These survival statistics will certainly improve as surgeons become more skilled. You'll find much more information about increasing your chances of survival in Chapter 9.

CHAPTER 6

Kidney and Pancreas Transplants

THIS CHAPTER DISCUSSES WHAT SORT OF PEOPLE will be considered for kidney, pancreas, and kidney-pancreas transplants, and it describes what happens before, during, and after surgery.

It's important to realize that different transplant teams have different ways of doing things. Depending on where you have your transplant done, some of the details presented in the following pages may vary.

While the chapter focuses on issues specific to kidney and pancreas recipients, it contains information of interest to the recipients of other transplants as well. Likewise, kidney and pancreas recipients may find relevant material in Chapters 4 and 5, which focus on heart, lung, and liver transplants. Although the details of the transplant surgeries themselves are obviously different, all transplant patients, no matter what organ they receive, share a good many common experiences. This is particularly true of post-surgical experiences, and you will want to peruse those sections of all three chapters.

Who gets kidney and pancreas transplants?

The main job of the kidneys is to filter waste material out of the blood, producing urine for excretion. In so doing, the kidneys help regulate blood volume, blood pressure, and the levels of sodium, potassium, and calcium in your body.

There are many diseases that can cause the kidneys to fail. When they do, the kidneys don't filter waste material properly, and these wastes build up in the body, a condition called uremia. Renal failure used to be uniformly and rapidly fatal, but since the invention of renal dialysis, people can be kept alive for many years despite having kidneys that do not function.

There are two types of dialysis—hemodialysis and peritoneal dialysis. Both are imperfect solutions to kidney failure, but they are effective in filtering wastes out of the body. Hemodialysis requires going to a dialysis center several times a week and being hooked up to a dialysis machine for up to four hours at a time. Peritoneal dialysis involves surgery to implant a catheter in the patient's belly. The patient must then dialyze herself several times a day (sometimes this can be done overnight) while taking great pains to avoid infection. People on both types of dialysis have to eat a special, highly restrictive diet.

Kidneys have other jobs besides filtering the blood. They also produce a number of hormones with important functions such as stimulating the production of red blood cells and regulating blood pressure. Dialysis cannot compensate for this loss of function. Therefore, the closest thing to a cure for kidney failure is a transplant.

Donald C. Dafoe, MD, director of Adult Kidney and Pancreas Transplant Programs at Stanford University Medical Center, describes who may be a candidate for kidney transplant:

> People who have renal failure and are on dialysis are candidates. The great, great majority—95 plus percent—are on dialysis already. But you might also do a pre-emptive kidney transplant for people who have renal insufficiency—they have not yet been dialyzed, but it's going to happen in the next few months.

Dr. Dafoe also discusses whether transplant or dialysis would be the treatment of choice:

> There used to be a kind of battle—which is better, dialysis or transplant? That's gone away. Transplant is the treatment of choice for renal failure. The problem is there's this huge organ shortage. So we see dialysis and transplant as complementary. But if someone is a reasonable candidate and they want a transplant, that is the goal now of the whole medical community. It's much more cost effective too. From the patient's point of view, they are much better rehabilitated. They're more independent. They're stronger.

> There's a mortality in the first year of dialysis of roughly 15 percent. For diabetics, it's 25 percent. Then it's also a deteriorative state. You have to restrict your protein. It's a sort of semi-starvation. It's hard on the body. Not to say that transplant is not, because of the drugs. But if you have a

room of transplant patients and a room of chronic dialysis patients, the difference smacks you in the face. Transplant patients are robust. The dialysis patients are sallow and tired looking.

Despite that, kidney transplants are not right for everyone with kidney disease. The transplant versus dialysis decision is one that must be made individually by each patient, in partnership with his or her physician. Even patients who are doing well with dialysis may desire to pursue a transplant. One reason for this is that someone on peritoneal dialysis may experience an infection that would render him unable to continue on dialysis. Another element that should enter into the decision is that the results of kidney transplants tend to be better if they're performed early in the course of the disease, before the ravages of kidney failure result in a weak and debilitated patient.

Diabetes is an inability of the body to properly digest sugars, and it's caused by a lack of the hormone insulin, which is produced in the pancreas. Many diabetics give themselves daily insulin injections and must keep a close eye on their diets and blood-sugar levels. As Dr. Dafoe explains, some diabetics are candidates for pancreas or kidney-pancreas transplants:

> *Anyone who gets a pancreas has to be a Type 1 diabetic, which is also called juvenile diabetes or insulin-dependent diabetes. The typical situation is that a child at age thirteen will come to the emergency room with a high blood-sugar level and will be diagnosed with Type 1 diabetes and prescribed insulin. Typically they go along for about twenty years, but when they're in their thirties, that's when the renal failure and other problems, such as eye problems, begin to manifest in a big way.*

> *In that setting, when the kidneys are gone, we will put in a kidney and pancreas from the same cadaver donor at the same time. That will normalize their sugars, maybe stave off the continued complications, and also replace their damaged kidneys. You might ask, why not put a pancreas in before the damage? Why not do it earlier? Well, the downside is immunosuppression. Most people think that a pancreas transplant alone prior to kidney failure is not successful enough. There's a big enough downside, both surgically and with chronic immunosuppression, that it's not warranted.*

People with Type II diabetes—also called adult-onset diabetes—are not candidates for pancreas transplants. Unfortunately, Type II diabetes is far more common than Type I.

Kidney transplants are the most common transplants performed. In the US in 1998, there were 11,990 kidney transplants, 253 pancreas transplants, and 965 combined kidney-pancreas transplants.

Qualifying for a kidney transplant

Not everyone with kidney failure is a candidate for a kidney transplant. If you're referred as a potential candidate for transplant, the transplant team will conduct a number of medical tests to ensure that you need a kidney and that you'll be likely to survive the operation. Although some of the qualifying criteria can seem harsh in individual cases, transplant teams focus on what will work. They want to maximize the results from a precious and scarce resource—donated organs—and make sure that a life will be saved.

One thing to remember is that not all transplant teams use the same criteria. If one medical center decides that you are not a candidate for transplant, you may want to investigate whether you might have access to other medical centers that use a somewhat different set of standards.

One way to increase your chances of qualifying for transplant is to find a living kidney donor. As explained in Chapter 2, *The System*, and in Chapter 13, *Living Donors*, someone who may be a marginal transplant candidate can often tip the scales in favor of transplant if a compatible relative—or even a friend—is willing to be a donor. Chapter 13 lists the many other advantages of living donation, one of the most significant of which is a greatly decreased waiting time.

As explained in Chapter 2, whether you'll be listed for a transplant depends on both medical and non-medical criteria. As Dr. Dafoe explains, in addition to conducting a thorough examination of your medical condition, the team will also evaluate your personality and your track record in managing your own health:

> We want people who are good stewards of their organs, and we want people who are going to show up for their appointments and take their medications. The best indication is their track record on dialysis and with their referring doctor. So our social worker talks to the dialysis social workers. If we hear they don't show up for dialysis, and then they show up in the emergency room two days later in fluid overload, and we have to dialyze them on an emergency basis, and when we talk to them they say they were on a bender or something like that, then that would

*obviously not be good. But it's a tough call, and there are people who hate
dialysis, and they behave very non-compliantly on dialysis. Then they get
a kidney and they say, "I don't want to jeopardize this," and they become
perfect patients. So we rely on our social workers and on our own gut
feelings after years and years of interviewing these candidates.*

*But active drug abuse or active alcoholism? They're out. Coronary
artery disease excludes them because the surgery is too risky. Other
exclusions include active HIV infection, and certain other active
infections.*

Dr. Dafoe points out, however, that exclusions based on HIV infections are
being re-evaluated based on the success of protease inhibitors and other
drugs that help control the virus.

While different transplant teams require different sets of medical tests during the evaluation procedure, almost every candidate is subjected to the following three tests:

- **Chest x-ray.** This helps rule out cancer. Cancers tend to spread rapidly
  when people are immunosuppressed, so people with cancer are generally not considered good transplant candidates.

- **Electrocardiogram.** This test examines the electrical activity of your
  heart, and can help determine whether you have any heart problems.

- **Blood tests.** Your blood will be tested for many different things. Your
  blood and tissue types will be determined this way, and your blood
  chemistry and your immune system will be evaluated. You'll also be
  tested for AIDS and other blood-borne diseases.

Depending on your medical condition and the practices of your transplant
team, you may also be subjected to some of the following additional tests:

- **Bone survey and hand x-ray.** These are tests for bone disease.

- **Upper gastrointestinal x-ray.** This determines whether you have an
  ulcer.

- **Lower gastrointestinal x-ray.** This test uses a barium enema to determine if you have any abnormalities in your intestines.

- **Gallbladder x-ray.** This determines whether you have gallstones.

- **Kidney tomogram.** This is an x-ray that allows your physician to determine the three-dimensional structure of your kidneys.

- **Pulmonary function test.** This tests the capacity of your lungs.

- **Cystoscopy.** A small fiber-optic cable will be inserted into your urethra so doctors can see your bladder. This test is normally conducted under general anesthesia.

- **Voiding cystourethrogram.** A catheter is inserted into your urethra, and a dye is injected into your bladder. As you urinate, x-ray photographs are taken to determine whether there are any abnormalities in your urinary tract.

- **Urodynamic study.** This test measures your bladder's capacity, its sensitivity, and your pattern of urination.

- **Sonogram.** This test uses sound waves to visualize the kidneys and surrounding structures.

One blood test you'll want to pay close attention to is your creatinine level, as it provides a direct measure of kidney function. Creatinine is an end-product of the digestion of food, and it is normally filtered out by the kidneys and excreted in the urine. When the kidneys are not functioning properly, elevated levels of creatinine will be found in the blood. Your doctors will keep a close eye on your creatinine both before and after transplant.

After transplant, a falling creatinine level will be one of the first indications that your new kidney is functioning properly. An increasing creatinine level, on the other hand, may be an early indication of rejection or of damage to the new kidney as an unfortunate side effect of immunosuppressive medication.

Unlike many other types of transplants, age is normally not a critical consideration in kidney transplants. These transplants are routinely performed on people in their seventies, especially when their physiological age is lower than their chronological age.

One thing to remember during the entire evaluation process is that unlike other transplant recipients, potential kidney recipients have the luxury of deciding whether or not to have transplant surgery. People who are in heart failure or who have end-stage liver disease are going to die without a transplant. This is not generally true of people with kidney disease. Many people live for decades on dialysis, and for some that may be a better solution that going in for major surgery, followed by a lifetime of powerful immunosuppressive medications. This is a decision that you should make carefully, in consultation with physicians, family members, and other medical and spiritual advisors.

Qualifying for pancreas transplants

Depending on the transplant team, potential pancreas and kidney-pancreas recipients will typically be subject to most or all of the same tests as are kidney recipients. But as kidney-pancreas recipient Lori Noyes points out, age is definitely a consideration in kidney-pancreas transplants. On top of that, she explains, diabetics with kidney disease have a more complicated choice—whether to have a kidney transplant alone or a kidney-pancreas transplant:

> I knew that kidney-pancreas transplants can only be done on people a certain age, and after 50 you're too old to get one. And I also knew I had a very healthy heart and circulation, which a lot of diabetics don't have. If I didn't go for a kidney-pancreas transplant now, if I didn't at least try, I would never ever forgive myself for not trying to be free of insulin. Also, a friend of mine told me a story of a guy who felt pressured to accept just a kidney because he was so ill. He was offered a kidney first, because it just happened to come up on the list, so he took it because kidney failure is what makes you sicker. We diabetics have lived without a functioning pancreas our whole lives. But to this day he has depression and anger over the fact that he never tried for the pancreas, and he's had problems with the kidney. I swore I would never do that to myself. I'm not going to live with the fact that I could have gone for both. I thought, "I have to try for it. If I reject it, fine, but at least I tried."

> Once I was on the list I had one false alarm. They called me six weeks into the wait and said, "We have a six out of six match kidney—a perfect match." It just hardly ever happens from a cadaver donor. They said, "Do you want it?" I said, "Well, you do have the pancreas with it don't you?" They said, "No. We called your nephrologist and he said you're really sick, and you should probably have the kidney," and that's when my trigger went off and I said, "No, no, no. Give it to someone else. I've been waiting years for a kidney and a pancreas. I want the package deal." They thought I was insane for turning it down, but a month later I got my kidney-pancreas transplant.

> Another nice benefit to a kidney-pancreas transplant is you have to get a very fresh, young, healthy, viable organ. They're called "pristine." My surgeon explained, "You get kind of a bonus here. You get a very short waiting time by getting both organs. Your waiting will be a year or less." He said the organs have to be pristine because the pancreas has to be

transplanted within about twelve or sixteen hours. Kidneys can wait seventy-two hours, but because you're getting both they're both going to be very young.

You'll find Lori's own account of her transplant experience at *http://www.geocities.com/HotSprings/2784/story1.html.*

Pancreas or kidney-pancreas transplants almost always come from a cadaveric donor. Some surgeons, however, are experimenting with living-donor pancreas transplants. A small part of a person's pancreas can be removed from a donor and implanted into a recipient. At this writing, living-donor pancreas transplants are still highly experimental, and are being performed by only a small number of transplant teams.

The surgery

If your kidney is coming from a living donor, both you and the donor will be admitted to the hospital about a day or two before surgery. But if you're waiting for a cadaveric kidney to become available, you'll be phoned or paged at some random moment, and asked to come into the hospital immediately. Once you get that call, don't eat or drink anything at all, since the surgeons prefer that you have a completely empty stomach during the operation.

While you're on the way in, a team from your hospital will be on its way to the donor to retrieve the organ. Working in cooperation with other teams from other hospitals there to retrieve the heart, liver, and other organs, your team will remove the donor's kidney. They will flush it out with a preservative solution, and then they'll attach a small pump to the kidney, intended to keep the preservative solution flowing. The kidney and pump are placed into a plastic bag, and that is placed into an ordinary picnic cooler filled with ice and preservative solution.

In this way, kidneys can be maintained for up to 72 hours before they're too old to transplant. That's the longest survival time of any transplanted organ. Nevertheless, it's always better to get a kidney that's been deprived of its blood supply for as short a time as possible.

When the kidney arrives at your hospital, you'll be prepped for surgery. You'll be anesthetized, and your abdomen will be shaved and washed with an iodine disinfectant solution. A Foley catheter will be inserted in your urethra to drain urine from your bladder.

Then the actual surgery starts. As Dr. Dafoe explains, kidney-transplant surgery is routine, and it doesn't take very long:

> *The kidney transplant is perhaps the most common operation done here. At Stanford it's more common than appendectomy. It's not really a big deal anymore. Kidney transplant surgery is routine and straightforward. I would say the degree of difficulty is 7 on a scale of 0 to 10, with pancreas being a 9 and a liver being 10. A typical kidney surgery takes three hours, but with pancreas surgery it's more like six hours.*

One thing it's important to know about kidney-transplant surgery is that in most cases your old kidneys will not be removed unless they are infected (or in some cases of polycystic kidney disease). Even in those cases, it's more common for the old kidneys to be removed in a separate operation that may take place months before—or months after—the transplant.

The kidneys normally are located deep in the lower abdomen, close to your back, on either side of the spine. Instead of putting the new kidney in that same spot, surgeons find it easier to place it in the front part of the abdominal cavity, cradled by your pelvic bone. Most commonly, the kidney is placed on your left side, but occasionally it'll be placed on the right. In Dave Souza's case, for example, he had had the catheter for peritoneal dialysis placed on the left, so the surgeons put his new kidney on the right.

The surgeon will make an incision above your groin. It'll be eight to ten inches long and angled like a hockey stick. In transplanting the new kidney, the surgeon has to make three anastomoses (connections). He has to connect the kidney's artery and vein to an artery and vein in your body, and he also has to connect the kidney's ureter, through which urine flows. There are two ways he can connect the ureter, and surgeons select the method based on their preference and on the details of your individual anatomy. He can choose to connect the ureter to one of the ureters from one of your old kidneys, or he can connect it directly to your bladder.

If you are receiving a pancreas instead of—or in addition to—a kidney, different surgeons will make different types of incisions. Some make two incisions of the type used in kidney transplants, one on either side of the lower abdomen. Others make a single incision down the middle of the abdomen, from above the belly button to the pubic bone. As with a kidney transplant, three connections have to be made. The new organ's vein and artery need to be connected to a vein and an artery in your body. This is the route through which insulin will flow. Once the vein and artery are hooked up, the pancreatic duct, which carries digestive secretions from the pancreas, has to be connected to something. In nature, the pancreatic duct is connected to your intestines, but many surgeons prefer not to connect the transplanted duct to your intestines, because cutting into the intestines carries a great risk of spreading infection. Instead, they'll connect the duct directly to your bladder, and the pancreas's digestive juices will be excreted with your urine. This provides the added benefit of allowing your doctor to monitor the health of the transplanted pancreas by performing simple urine tests. Other surgeons, however, do prefer to connect the pancreatic duct to the small bowel, and this type of surgery is becoming more common.

Once the organ or organs are transplanted, your incision will be sewn or stapled closed, and you'll be taken to the recovery room.

Immediately after surgery

Once you're in the recovery room, you'll gradually awaken. You may find that there's a tube in your throat and that you're connected to a ventilator, a machine that's breathing for you. More commonly, though, the tube and the ventilator will have been removed before you awaken.

It's likely that you'll experience some pain, although the amount of pain experienced by Lori Noyes after her kidney-pancreas surgery is somewhat unusual:

> The surgery itself took approximately eight hours. Then I was in the recovery room for a couple of hours. When I woke up, I remember yelling because I was in a lot of pain. I wasn't very pretty when I came out. My mom said they could hear me all the way down the hallway. The pain was from the incision, and it only lasted a couple of days. I don't think the tubes bothered me. I just remember saying, "I can't breathe. I can't get enough air in." I didn't have a respirator, but I could not catch enough air. It may have been more mental than actual, because they said I was fine. I was on oxygen—I had it in my nose. But for some reason I could not catch my breath.

> My mom said I was obnoxious when I came out from surgery. I remember a few hours later the whole team of doctors came in, and they were all grinning from ear to ear, and I was of course in just a miserable,

miserable mood. They came in and said, "How are you?" I said, "Awful. What do you want?" They said, "We're just here to tell you your transplant was a great success. Your kidney and pancreas have already started working and we're just so pleased about that." I said, "That's wonderful," not really meaning it. It wasn't until I learned about transplants that I found out that it's a big deal to have the kidney work right away, because sometimes it sleeps for a while. And the pancreas—my blood sugars were still around 200, and I thought that was high, and they said, "But you're not taking insulin, so that's pretty good. If you were truly a diabetic and not on insulin, it should have been 800." So that was proof that the pancreas was working.

That day was horrible, and I don't lie to new people who are going to get a transplant. I say, "You won't feel all that great your first day."

Dave Souza apparently experienced pain just after surgery, but he remembers little of it. It's quite common for people waking from surgery to have entire conversations that they don't remember the next day:

Some nurse came in to me the next morning and said, "Oh, you're the guy who was yelling, 'I'd give a dollar for being any other place but here!'" but I have no recollection of that. The first thing I do remember is Linda being by the bed and talking to me and stuff. And then after that the doctors came in. That's when I found out everything went fine. There was no pain, basically. I was pretty mellow. And I think it was either then or after they let me sleep a little bit longer, but they wanted me up on my feet, just to take a few steps, away from the bed and then back. I noticed I couldn't move, I wasn't flexible. I was very weak-footed. And then I slept again.

They get you up and moving around very quickly. They're very intent on that, every morning. And after two or three mornings, I was intent on making laps, walking around the entire corridor of that one ward. I think twelve laps was a mile, six laps was a half-mile.

Recovery

As you recover in the hospital, your doctors will be eager to see how your new organs are functioning. As Dave Souza reports, they took an intense interest in the volume, color, and composition of his urine:

> *They were all coming in looking at my urine, like they thought I was a brewery or something: "Oh, look at the color," they would say, and they were happy with it from the beginning.*

Dave Souza found that he experienced only moderate pain, which was easily alleviated by Vicodin, a relatively mild narcotic pain pill:

> *They always asked me, "How's your pain, on a 1 to 10 scale?" And I never felt any worse than a 5 or a 6, and it wasn't really pain, it was just discomfort. It was my abdomen, basically. The more I was there, the more I felt where the sutures were. The area where my new kidney was felt bruised for a few weeks if not a whole month afterward. After the major anesthetic wore off I was on an IV drip of pain medication for four days. Then I was just on Vicodin by request. If I said I had pain, then they would give me Vicodin. At night I would ask for one and the nurse would say, "Would you like two?" and I'd say, "No, just one to help me sleep," because it just made me comfortable enough to where I wasn't fidgeting through the night.*

After a few days, they'll remove the Foley catheter, which can be an uncomfortable experience. The Foley catheter is a thin tube that's inserted up the urethra into the bladder. Once it's in the bladder a small balloon around the end of the tube in the bladder is inflated with saline solution. This prevents the Foley from slipping out accidentally. When it's time to remove the Foley, the balloon is deflated and the entire catheter is pulled out. Some people report that they can feel the spot where the balloon had been for several days after the catheter is removed. As Dave Souza puts it:

> *The one uncomfortable part about the whole hospital stay, though, was when they took out the Foley catheter, three or four days after the surgery. I was very friendly with my Foley. It didn't bother me at all until the day they pulled it out. It was an unusual feeling. It really wasn't painful. The length of that sucker that was hidden in me was amazing. Then they wanted me to make sure I urinated at least once every half hour so I wouldn't expand my bladder. So that meant I went that first night without sleep after they pulled out the Foley.*

You'll be started on immunosuppressives immediately after—and sometimes even just before—surgery. At first the dose will be very high, but it will gradually decline.

The amount of time a patient remains in the hospital depends on what type of surgery he received. After a living related kidney transplant, the length of stay is normally five days. After a cadaveric transplant, it can be eight days. For kidney-pancreas recipients, everything's longer and more elaborate, and the length of stay can be ten to twelve days.

But if there are complications, such as an infection, you may be in the hospital longer. That's what happened to Lori Noyes:

> I was in the hospital for three weeks, and I said, "Send me home." So they did even though I was still running a temperature once in a while. I went home with home nursing, but within three days I was readmitted with a high fever and a cough. They never did figure out what was wrong with me. It was probably a respiratory infection. It was not a rejection episode, and it was not a major infection, which was good. They gave me a blood transfusion and antibiotics for a week, and then I was fine.

> But I didn't feel well. I felt like I was hit by a truck for the first two months. I was still sleeping a lot, and feeling wiped out. I was kind of impatient, and the doctor said, "You had major surgery. It could take six months before you feel human again." But two months after the surgery it was almost an overnight sensation where I woke up one day feeling really good and energetic, and I thought, "Wow, this is a great day! I feel like exercising. I feel like going outside." And I did. Then I started walking on a treadmill we had in the house. I was still using a cane and all that, but I felt great, and I couldn't figure out why. I know one part of it was that the prednisone had been tapered enough where I was feeling better mentally—no longer depressed.

Six months after his transplant, Dave Souza was feeling practically normal, although he still experiences some tenderness around his incision:

> I've been wearing suspenders a lot, and I still can't wear a belt. I still notice my sutures at work when I do lifting. I'm trying to stay within a 50-pound weight limit, but as a furniture salesman, we have to do the stocking and the loading of customers' cars and things like that.

CHAPTER 7

Other Transplants

UP TO NOW WE'VE LIMITED OUR DISCUSSION to the most common solid-organ transplants. But there are a number of tissues and organs aside from hearts, lungs, livers, kidneys, and pancreases that can be transplanted, and we'll devote this chapter to those other transplants.

Some of these transplants are extremely common. Transplant of the cornea is the most common transplant operation performed in the US. Others, such as bone-marrow transplants, are becoming an increasingly routine part of medical care. Still others, such as whole-limb transplants, remain highly experimental and highly controversial.

Corneas

The cornea is the clear outer covering at the front of the eye. Its precise curvature is responsible for focusing light onto the retina. There are a number of conditions and diseases that can damage the cornea. Anything that causes the cornea to become scarred, cloudy, or irregular in shape will interfere with vision. These include:

- Various hereditary conditions, such as keratoconus and Fuchs' dystrophy

- Infections, such as herpes

- Corneal failure as an accidental side effect of other eye surgery

- Injury, such as damage from a foreign body or caustic chemicals

More than 45,000 corneal transplants are performed in the US each year. This is more than all solid-organ transplants combined. Corneal transplants have a very long history as well. The first one was performed back in 1905.

Corneal transplants are performed by ophthalmologists. Most are performed as outpatient surgery in a hospital. The ophthalmologist may choose to use local or general anesthesia, depending on the recipient's age, medical condition, and eye disease.

In the first step, the old cornea is removed by an instrument called a trephine, which is something like a cookie cutter. The donor cornea is then sewn on with a very fine thread that will stay in the eye for months or even years as the cornea heals.

The recipient is almost always sent home on the same day as the surgery. Post-transplant treatment typically involves nothing more than eye drops that must be placed in the eye several times a day. These medications will typically include a topical steroid to ward off rejection.

Rejection is usually not a major problem after corneal transplants, and the topical steroid is usually all that's required to prevent its appearance. However, 20 percent of cornea recipients do show signs of rejection. These signs include persistent discomfort, light sensitivity, redness, or a change in vision. Rejection is usually treated successfully with a course of systemic immunosuppressive therapy.

Until recently it was thought that there was no need to match the blood type or tissue type of the donor cornea to the recipient (see Chapter 3, *The Wait*, for more on blood and tissue matching). However, recent studies have suggested that people at high risk for rejection (such as those who have previously rejected a cornea) are less likely to experience rejection if blood types—but not tissue types—are matched. These studies remain controversial.

All corneas for transplantation come from cadaveric donors. The procurement and distribution of corneas is handled by a set of local organizations called eye banks. All eye banks in the US are members of UNOS.

In several states, the rules for cornea donations are somewhat different than the rules for organ donations. Some states permit eye banks to remove corneas from recently deceased individuals without obtaining permission from the donor's family, as long as neither the family nor the donor has specifically objected to such donations. Occasionally the donor family is not even informed that their loved one's corneas have been taken. This sometimes causes hard feelings and controversy when such policies come to light.

Corneas need not be removed while the donor remains on life support. They remain viable even several hours after respiration and blood circulation have ceased. Therefore, even people who are not eligible to donate any other organs may be able to give the gift of sight to someone else.

In addition, corneas need not be transplanted immediately. With modern preservative solutions, corneas can remain viable for up to ten days after they have been removed from donors.

Since so many corneas are available, people needing corneas typically have a very short wait for transplant.

For more on corneal transplants, contact the Eye Bank Association of America at (202) 775-4999 or online at *http://www.restoresight.org/*. (You'll find full contact information in the appendix, *Resources*.)

Small intestine

Partially digested food from the stomach enters the small intestine, a long tube in which additional digestion takes place, and from which nutrients are absorbed into the bloodstream. In adults the small intestine is about 23 feet long. Waste material passes from the small intestine to the much shorter (but wider) large intestine for elimination.

The small intestine can become damaged in several ways. Blood clots, injury, Crohn's disease, or other inflammatory bowel diseases can result in the loss of large sections of the small intestine. If more than 70 percent of the small intestine is lost, the result is "short-gut syndrome."

People with short-gut syndrome cannot properly digest their food, so they are not permitted to take any food by mouth. They must receive all their nutrition via a tube permanently implanted in a large vein in the chest. This is referred to as total parenteral nutrition (TPN). People on TPN frequently must remain connected to a machine for 12 hours a day.

Until recently, people with short-gut syndrome could expect to get all of their nutrition via TPN for the rest of their lives. But beginning in the late 1980s, surgeons began performing transplants of the small intestine. Sometimes the small intestine is transplanted alone, sometimes it is transplanted together with the liver, and sometimes it is transplanted together with the liver, pancreas, and stomach. Almost half of all intestine recipients are children.

Successful intestine transplants allow recipients to return to a normal life and to eat solid food. For some, this is the first time in many years that they have been able to do so.

At first, survival rates were not very impressive. In the early years of intestinal transplants, only about 35 percent of recipients survived more than a year. But greater surgical experience and new immunosuppressive drugs are resulting in steadily improving survival times. A UNOS study of all intestinal transplants in the US between 1987 and 1997 found that 59.2 percent of grafts and 68.0 percent of recipients survived more than one year, and 35.0 percent of grafts and 45.0 percent of patients survived more than four years.

There are indications that survival times are continuing to increase. In May 1999, the University of Pittsburgh Medical Center, which performs about 40 percent of all intestinal transplants worldwide, announced that 92 percent of its most recent patients had survived for at least one year. Twenty-two of their 121 patients have so far survived more than five years, and one patient has survived more than nine years. However, a smaller proportion of grafts survive, and when the donor intestine is rejected the patient must return to TPN.

Intestine transplants are still relatively rare operations. Only 65 were performed in the US in 1997 and only 68 in 1998. As this is being written, 116 people are on the waiting list in the US for intestine transplants.

Whole limbs

The ability to transplant whole limbs has been a dream of surgeons for thousands of years. According to legend, the first physicians to succeed at this operation were the twin brothers, Saints Cosmos and Damian. The brothers, who were born in Arabia and died circa 283 AD, replaced the gangrenous leg of the Roman deacon Justinian with a leg from a recently buried Ethiopian Moor. This is referred to as "the miracle of the black leg." Cosmos and Damian are considered the patron saints of pharmacists.

Flash forward almost 1,700 years to the mid-1960s, when surgeons made several attempts to transplant hands or forearms. The longest-lived of these grafts survived only fourteen days, but that was an era before the discovery of effective immunosuppressants. In 1998 and 1999, surgeons in France and the US made two widely reported attempts to transplant whole limbs. In each case the recipients were individuals who had had an arm amputated below the elbow years before.

Limb transplants are highly complex operations. When a surgeon transplants a heart or a kidney, she need only make connections between a few blood vessels. In a whole-limb transplant, on the other hand, the surgeon must connect bone, muscle, tendons, nerves, and skin in addition to the blood vessels.

While each of the two arms has survived more than six months as of this writing, it's unclear how much function the recipients have regained. For the recipient to experience sensation or to regain fine motor control of the fingers requires that the recipient's nerves grow out into the graft. Even if the surgeon were successful in lining up the recipient's nerves with the donor's— a surgical feat that requires microscopic precision—one would expect the nerves to regrow only very slowly, perhaps a millimeter or two a month. Virtually no physicians, including the ones who performed these operations, expect the recipients ever to regain full muscular control or normal sensation.

Whole-limb transplants are exceedingly controversial. Critics of the procedure suggest that it violates the main principle of the Hippocratic Oath: "First, do no harm." Someone who has lost a limb can live a full life in good health, but a transplant can risk that person's good health in several ways. First of all, a limb transplant exposes a healthy person to the significant risks of surgery. A small percentage of people never awaken from general anesthesia, and surgery always carries with it the risk of infection and other complications. Secondly, the transplant recipient will have to take powerful immunosuppressive medications for the rest of his life. As described in Chapter 8, *Anti-Rejection Drugs*, and Chapter 9, *Living with a Transplant*, these drugs can have serious—even life-threatening—side effects. Finally, some argue that limb transplants are unnecessary, since modern prosthetic limbs can return a great deal of function to an amputee.

On the other hand, argue advocates of the procedure, it should be up to the potential recipient, in conjunction with his physician, to judge the level of risk that's acceptable. Some people who have lost a limb find that living without it is so inconvenient that they're willing to take a calculated risk. And if you accept the argument that limb transplants should be prohibited because prosthetics provide a reasonable level of functionality, then shouldn't kidney transplants be prohibited because dialysis does the same?

The ethical questions aside, it's too soon to tell whether whole-limb transplants will ever become more than rarely performed medical curiosities. Routine limb transplants are at minimum several years away.

Bone marrow

Bone marrow is a deep-red spongy material that normally resides within the hollow spaces of living bone. "Stem cells" within the bone marrow give rise to the major components of blood, including red blood cells, which carry oxygen to all the cells of the body; white blood cells, which as part of the immune system ward off infection; and platelets, which help the blood to clot.

Bone marrow is transplanted for a variety of reasons. Leukemia is a form of cancer in which the bone marrow's stem cells multiply uncontrollably, producing an excessive number of immature blood cells. Aplastic anemia is a condition in which the stem cells produce too few blood cells. In both conditions, replacing the defective bone marrow with healthy donor marrow can relieve the symptoms, at least temporarily and occasionally for long periods.

A bone marrow transplant (often abbreviated BMT) may also be useful for someone undergoing chemotherapy for other forms of cancer. Although this form of therapy is quite controversial, in an attempt to kill cancer cells, physicians often wish to administer high doses of relatively toxic medicines. While cancer cells are particularly susceptible to these toxic chemicals, so are bone marrow cells. Physicians used to be placed on the horns of a dilemma. They could either give low doses of chemotherapy to protect the bone marrow, but risk that some cancer cells would survive, or they could give high doses of chemotherapy to kill all the cancer cells, but risk that the patient's bone marrow would be destroyed as well. A person whose bone marrow has been destroyed will be extremely susceptible to infection, and also will develop a severe anemia, since his body won't be producing any blood cells.

Bone marrow transplantation may be an answer. If the patient's marrow is normal, it will be harvested and stored before the chemotherapy is administered, and then returned to the patient afterward. This situation, in which the patient is his own donor, is referred to as an autologous bone marrow transplant. If the patient's bone marrow is abnormal (as in leukemia or aplastic anemia), it may be subject to a process in which the abnormal cells are purged and the healthy cells are retained. This process, unfortunately, is imperfect, and an alternative is to use bone marrow from a matching donor. This is referred to as an allogeneic bone marrow transplant.

Allogeneic bone marrow transplants are highly susceptible to rejection and to graft-versus-host disease (GVHD) in which the transplanted marrow attacks the recipient's other cells. To avoid this, it's best if the marrow's donor has a tissue type that's a perfect six-of-six match with the recipient. (See Chapter 3 for more on tissue matching.) An individual has a 35 percent chance of having a brother or sister who's a perfect match. If no sibling matches, the next best alternative is to find a match among the many generous people who have signed up as potential donors with a national or international bone marrow registry.

Donating marrow involves little risk and only a small amount of discomfort. The harvesting of bone marrow generally takes place in a hospital operating room with the donor under general anesthesia. A long needle is inserted into the hip bone, which has a large supply of bone marrow. Several bone punctures on each hip will be required to remove the necessary amount of marrow. Depending on the size of the donor and the recipient's requirements, the physicians will withdraw about one to two quarts of blood and marrow. While this may seem like a lot, it's actually only about 2 percent of the body's total supply.

Once the anesthesia wears off, the donor will typically experience discomfort around the harvest sites that has been likened to that from a hard fall on the ice. The donor is usually discharged from the hospital the next day and can resume normal activities a few days later.

Bone marrow transplantation is highly complex, and has far too many ramifications to be explored fully in this short space. For more information, see the *Bone & Marrow Transplant Newsletter* and especially its handbook *Bone Marrow Transplants: a Book of Basics for Patients*, which is available by calling (888) 597-7674 or online at *http://www.bmtnews.org/*. Another good resource is *Bone Marrow Transplants: A Guide for Cancer Patients and Their Families,* by Marianne L. Shaffer, RN.

Other tissues

Many other body tissues can be transplanted for a wide variety of conditions. These tissues include:

- Heart valves
- Skin

- Ligaments

- Tendons

- Bone

- Major blood vessels

- Muscle covering (fascia)

The organizations responsible for procuring, processing, storing, and distributing tissue are called tissue banks. All tissue banks are accredited by the American Association of Tissue Banks: (703) 827-9582 or online at *http://www.aatb.org/*. American Red Cross Tissue Services is one of the largest tissue banks in the US, and it maintains an informative web site at *http://www.redcross.org/tissue/*.

More than 150,000 people each year receive donated tissue. The tissue is obtained from deceased or surgical donors who are tested for various diseases, including AIDS and hepatitis. Donated tissue is processed into almost 400 different forms. Some tissue is freeze dried, some is frozen, and some is fresh. Bone is often demineralized or powdered.

Among the many ways that this tissue is used are the following:

- Dental implants

- Replacement heart valves

- Treatment of burn injuries

- Replacement of bone lost due to injury or disease

- Plastic surgery

- Joint reconstruction

Tissue recipients virtually never have to worry about rejection and never need to take immunosuppressant medication. In fact, blood types need not be matched between donor and recipient. In most cases—such as with heart valves or bone—the treatment renders the tissue immunologically neutral, so the recipient's immune system doesn't recognize the material as foreign.

One exception to this is skin used with burn victims. In this case, the donor skin is used as sort of a scaffolding as the recipient's body slowly regenerates its own skin covering. The donor skin will eventually be rejected and will shrivel away, but by that time the recipient's skin will be well along in the regeneration process.

CHAPTER 8

Anti-Rejection Drugs

IF THERE'S ONE WORD every transplant recipient dreads, that word is "rejection." There's something particularly devastating about the thought that your own body is trying to kill a vital organ. Your body's immune system protects you by attacking anything it regards as foreign. This protects your health when infections or viruses threaten you with illness or when rogue cells from your own body threaten to grow out of control. When you are a transplant recipient, your body's natural defenses prevent you from incorporating and living with a foreign organ. To keep these defenses in check, you'll be taking anti-rejection drugs, usually in large amounts just after the transplant and on adjusted maintenance levels for the rest of your life. To give you the best quality of life, your medical team will be searching for just the right drugs at just the right dosages that protect you from the body's rejection response and that also minimize side effects.

In this chapter, we'll talk about what rejection is and how it is controlled. We'll go into a bit of detail on each of the standard immunosuppressive (anti-rejection) drugs, describing what they do and what side effects they may have. Finally we'll see how your transplant team would treat a rejection episode.

What rejection is

Taber's Cyclopedic Medical Dictionary (17th Edition, Philadelphia: F.A. Davis Company, 1993) defines rejection as the "destruction of transplanted material at the cellular level by the host's immune mechanism."

"Destruction . . . at the cellular level" sounds so final and so hopeless that it's important to remember is that in most cases rejection is not the end of the world. Since doctors are always trying to find the smallest dosage of anti-rejection drugs to do the job, often it's the early signs of rejection that tell doctors they have gone too low in dosage. While not all transplant patients will experience rejection, many do without suffering lasting ill effects. As heart-transplant recipient Jim Gleason writes,

> Rejection is really a good sign that the transplant team is aggressively trying to cut back on the steroids and other immune suppressant medications. This is very important since the body is open to attack by so many enemies while immune suppressed—a condition necessary to keep that same immune system from treating that "foreign" heart as an intruder and rejecting it. . . .
>
> Please don't underestimate the seriousness of rejection—without treatment it is fatal! When you experience your own rejection, don't get upset or worried, just do what the team prescribes and have trust in them. Listen to them carefully and report anything unusual for them to decide its importance.

To understand rejection, it's important to understand how the immune system works. You may wish to go back to Chapter 3, *The Wait*, and read the section "Finding a match," which discusses the immune system in the context of finding a matching organ.

There are three main kinds of rejection. The most severe is called hyperacute rejection. Somewhat less severe is acute rejection. Least severe is chronic rejection.

Hyperacute rejection is virtually instantaneous, and in the unlikely event that it happens, it's noticed during surgery, within minutes after the donor organ is placed in the recipient's body. If a recipient has a large number of antibodies in the bloodstream that react with the donor organ, there may be a hyperacute rejection. Recipients can acquire such antibodies in various ways. For example, transplant physicians would expect hyperacute rejection if the recipient's blood type is incompatible with the donor's. If the recipient has been sensitized by a transfusion, pregnancy, or a prior transplant, the bloodstream may carry antibodies that will react with the donor organ. The bad news about hyperacute rejection is that there is no treatment for it. The good news is that it's very rarely seen, because the transplant team makes sure blood types are compatible before anyone is ever brought to surgery, and they will test for sensitization.

Acute rejection is most likely to take place in the several weeks immediately following surgery, but it is also possible even years later. Acute rejection won't happen immediately, because it takes several days for the immune system's T cells to recognize the donor organ as foreign and to marshal a response. Immunosuppressive drugs are aimed squarely at preventing acute rejection. If these drugs weren't used, virtually all transplanted organs would be rejected within two weeks. The only exception would be organs transplanted between identical twins. Even with today's sophisticated anti-rejection strategies, many transplant patients will experience one or more episodes of acute rejection. While such episodes are serious and must be treated promptly and aggressively—normally by high doses of anti-rejection drugs administered during a hospital stay—in most cases acute rejection can be resolved satisfactorily.

Chronic rejection is a slow deterioration of the donor organ that takes place over a period of months to years. It's not well understood, and it's not well controlled by immunosuppressive medication either. Chronic rejection of a transplanted heart sometimes manifests itself as a slow deterioration of the heart muscle, or a progressive narrowing of the coronary arteries, which supply blood to the heart. Chronic rejection of a transplanted kidney results in an increase in creatinine levels.

As a transplant patient, you may not notice the symptoms of rejection before your doctor does. Some transplant recipients who are children may notice a fever. For kidney recipients, the symptoms of rejection can include swelling, decreased urine output, high blood pressure, graft tenderness, or weight gain. Heart recipients rarely notice any rejection symptoms, and liver recipients are unlikely to notice anything except, occasionally, for jaundice.

The important thing to realize is that you may be experiencing rejection even if you have no overt symptoms. That's why your doctor will insist on conducting regular tests. Depending on the type of transplant you've received, your doctor can diagnose rejection on the basis of blood tests, ultrasound exams, or biopsies before you feel any symptoms. This is an important reason not to begin skipping your regular clinic appointments even when you feel fine.

Keeping rejection in check

Most of the work of keeping rejection in check will fall to your transplant team as they monitor your body's response. Your own part in the process will be to take your medications religiously, to keep your clinic appointments scrupulously, to report any unusual symptoms, to become well informed about your condition, to keep good records, to alert other medical professionals to your history, and to be your own advocate. These and similar issues are covered in Chapter 9, *Living with a Transplant*.

To keep rejection in check, transplant researchers have developed a number of strategies using various anti-rejection drugs. All of these drugs have side effects, some of them unpleasant. During the course of their experience with transplants, physicians have determined that in most cases it's best to use a combination of drugs. If they used only one drug, they'd have to use high doses, and the result would be a high probability of bad side effects. By using a combination of drugs, the doses of each can be kept relatively low, so the side effects aren't as severe.

Still, physicians tend to start transplant patients on high doses of the drugs immediately after transplant, slowly reducing them as the patient recovers and shows no signs of rejection. Some physicians eventually eliminate some of the drugs entirely, but most physicians regard this as a dangerous practice and strongly advise against it. Almost all transplant patients should expect to be taking at least one—and sometimes several—immunosuppressive drugs for the rest of their lives.

One important thing to remember about immunosuppressive medication is that each patient is unique. Doses and combinations of these drugs have to be tailored individually. Some people will need only low doses, while others will need large amounts of the same medications. Some people will experience unacceptable side effects to one medication, and may have to be switched to another.

On top of that, finding the right combination of immunosuppressive drugs is more art than science. Different physicians and different transplant teams have different styles of treating their patients and different preferences for medications. You may meet another recipient in a support group or on the Internet who's doing very well taking some other combination of drugs than you are. This doesn't mean that you're getting second-class treatment.

On the other hand, don't be afraid to tell your doctor if you find some of the side effects of the drugs especially unpleasant. With the variety of immunosuppressive drugs available now—and with more due to come out of the pipeline in the near future—your doctor has greater flexibility than ever before in finding a combination that will work for you.

Here's what some transplant physicians have to say about their strategies and tactics in prescribing anti-rejection drugs. You'll notice that even physicians practicing at the same institution (all three quoted below are from Stanford University) have different styles of using these medications.

Emmet B. Keeffe, MD, Director of the Liver Transplant Program at Stanford University, describes his preference:

> *Different programs have different preferences for drugs. In our program, our preference is to use Prograf and prednisone. If there is a rejection episode we treat that and then we may add a third drug. We used to use Imuran, but now we more often use CellCept as the third drug.*

Donald C. Dafoe, MD, Director of Adult Kidney and Pancreas Transplant Programs at Stanford University, describes a somewhat different set of drugs preferred by his team:

> *For kidney recipients, we use so-called triple therapy: cyclosporine in the Neoral form, CellCept, and prednisone. Some people get FK506, but we still use that more as rescue if cyclosporine fails. For kidney-pancreas recipients, we use FK506, CellCept, and prednisone. These patients have a lot more rejection, and I think FK506 is a stronger anti-rejection drug than cyclosporine. It's just got different side effects.*
>
> *As the person gets healthier, they absorb the drugs better. So over time, you can lower the dose, particularly cyclosporine or FK506. But there does come a point where it's dangerous to continue to lower doses. At some point, maybe at the end of a year, they're on maintenance and that's where they're going to live. Some groups taper prednisone off because steroids do have a lot of side effects. But virtually every study I know demonstrates that you pay a price for that, so we don't do it as a general policy. Occasionally there are compelling reasons to get rid of one drug or another, and then you tailor it to the patient as best you can. Occasionally a patient will come in and they'll confess that they haven't taken their drugs for a year and they're doing fine. So it's clear there are some people that don't need it after a while. But the overall experience of a non-compliant patient is very bad. They usually lose their grafts and sometimes their lives. We can't distinguish which ones will do poorly and which ones won't.*

Sharon A. Hunt, MD, a cardiologist at Stanford University, describes her program's desire to wean patients from prednisone:

> We try to get patients down to a fairly low dose of prednisone within the first six months, and then after that we select our candidates for getting off steroids. Those who haven't had any rejection have a decent chance for getting off. We get lots of our patients off, I'd guess 20 to 25 percent.

Your medications

The drugs used to suppress your body's immune response are strong ones. Because they suppress such a basic bodily function, they can cause many side effects. Even if your side effects are very slight, it is always a good idea to know about the drugs you are taking, what symptoms to call to your doctors' attention, and what alternatives might be available.

The drugs described here (in rough order of frequency of use among transplant patients) include:

- Prednisone and other steroids
- Neoral and Sandimmune (cyclosporine)
- Prograf (tacrolimus)
- Imuran (azathioprine)
- CellCept (mycophenolate mofetil)
- Rapamune (sirolimus)
- Other medications (to control side effects)

For each drug, we'll say a little about its mode of action, and then we'll describe potential side effects.

Prednisone and other steroids

Almost every transplant patient takes prednisone (or one of its relatives), and this is the drug almost every transplant patient learns to hate. Despite side effects that can be unpleasant, prednisone is virtually unmatched in its ability to suppress the immune system.

Prednisone is sold under the trade names Deltasone, Cortan, and Orasone, (among others) but is also available in generic versions. It is an artificial glucocorticoid. Your body makes natural glucocorticoids such as cortisol in your adrenal glands, which sit atop your kidneys. Chemically speaking, the molecular structure of glucocorticoids classifies them as steroids, but they should not be confused with the anabolic steroids—like the male sex hormone testosterone—which some athletes take to put on muscle mass. The natural function of the glucocorticoids is to protect the body against stress and to assist in protein and carbohydrate metabolism.

Prednisone and related drugs are prescribed for a wide variety of conditions. In addition to immunosuppression for transplant patients, these drugs are used to reduce inflammation and for a wide variety of other conditions such as asthma, allergies, endocrine disorders, and rheumatoid arthritis.

Depending on your medical condition and your doctor's preference, you may be prescribed not prednisone but another closely related compound. The most common alternatives to prednisone are prednisolone (trade names Cortalone and Delta-Cortef) and methylprednisolone (Medrol). The list below contains the generic names of the most commonly used glucocorticoids. All of these compounds have similar actions and similar side effects. Since prednisone is the one most commonly prescribed for transplant patients, that's the one we'll discuss most directly, but almost everything we say about prednisone will apply to whatever steroid you have been prescribed.

Here's a list of the generic names of other glucocorticoids used on occasion for immunosuppression:

- Beclomethosone
- Cortisone acetate
- Dexamethasone
- Fludrocortisone acetate
- Hydrocortisone
- Methyprednisolone
- Paramethasone acetate
- Prednisolone
- Prednisone
- Triamcinolone

Dosage

Steroid dosages vary from person to person, and your dose will also vary over time. You'll probably be given fairly high doses of steroids in the hospital immediately after your transplant. In the hospital these doses are typically delivered intravenously, using a form of methyprednisolone called Solu-Medrol. You may very well be started at an IV dose of 100 to 200 mg (milligrams) per day, but that will be tapered off rapidly. By the time you leave the hospital, you'll be taking prednisone in pill form.

Kidney recipient Dave Souza talks about how his prednisone was reduced:

> After the hospital they started me off at 80 mg, and then they tapered it off. Well, they tapered it too fast, and the week before Thanksgiving I started showing signs of a rejection. So they put me back in the hospital for three days and they put me on a prednisone drip of almost 200 mg a day. Then when I left they put me up to 180 mg in pills a day, and now I'm down to 7.5 mg a day. But I've kept my salt down, I've kept my sugar down, and that's why I don't have the Charlie Brown head like a lot of people on prednisone do.

If you show evidence of rejection, you'll often be readmitted to the hospital where you'll be given high-dose steroids intravenously. We'll discuss this in more detail later in this chapter, in the section "Treating rejection."

Physical side effects

The "Charlie Brown head" that Dave mentions earlier is one of the common side effects of prednisone. One's face tends to swell, giving people on prednisone a characteristic round, moon face, like the cartoon character in the Peanuts strip. Because of this characteristic, Melanie Horne can pick out other transplant patients by sight:

> My face has certainly changed. It's kind of funny because all transplant patients can recognize each other by the chipmunk cheeks. You'll run into somebody, and you'll say, "You've had a transplant, haven't you?" "How'd you know?" "Oh, I get it, you haven't seen yourself in the mirror yet, have you?" Yeah, your face changes.

Prednisone also tends to make people hungry. This is a welcome improvement for some liver transplant patients, since they may have suffered from poor appetite for several years. Once they've been transplanted they find that they're ravenous and want to eat everything.

The prednisone munchies make it very easy to put on far too much weight far too quickly. Many transplant patients gain thirty to eighty pounds in a matter of months. For this reason, you will most likely be told to watch your weight very carefully, and to eat a low-fat, low-salt diet. Jim Gleason had that experience:

> The weight gain is an ongoing struggle, driven by the hunger generated by those steroids. Everything that fats and cholesterol can do to the "normal" person is magnified by the steroids in the transplanted patient, so the danger of clogged arteries, etc., is much greater. Thus my diet is low-everything!

The extra weight from prednisone tends to be distributed oddly. Weight tends to accumulate in the belly and in the upper back, which can make people seem round-shouldered or slightly hunched. On the other hand, people on prednisone tend to have skinny legs and skinny arms.

Other physical side effects of prednisone include elevated blood pressure, elevated cholesterol, and stomach problems. Taking prednisone with meals may help alleviate the stomach upset.

Kidney-pancreas recipient Lori Noyes has experienced many of prednisone's physical side effects:

> Four months after I left the hospital the blood pressure went up, the cholesterol went up, the hair started growing, my legs got skinny, my abdomen got bigger, and my arms got skinny. It's typical—I can point out steroid patients on any street corner because of that look that we all have.

Psychological side effects

The physical side effects, disturbing as they may be to people concerned about their appearance, tend not to be the most bothersome reactions to prednisone. Steroids—especially at the high doses you'll be taking soon after the transplant or a rejection episode—can cause a variety of psychological reactions as well. These can range from mildly annoying—irritability, restlessness, depression, and mood swings, for example—to quite frightening—vivid hallucinations are not unusual. The more severe psychological reactions tend to occur at the very high doses given in the hospital, and not at lower maintenance doses. Lori Noyes had a typical high-dose response:

> I was having a lot of mental effects from the drugs. They were giving me tons of steroids—IV Solu-Medrol, which is a form of prednisone. They

told me it was a couple hundred milligrams, but it is instantly tapered down. I was having insomnia, nightmares, vivid dreams, and depression, and I couldn't figure out where that was coming from. It was evident in my mood that something was wrong, but the nurses didn't know me, and none of them bothered to just say something to me like, "The prednisone can do this to you."

I was pretty witchy. I remember a couple of ICU nurses saying, "You need to calm down." I remember thinking, "What is with me?" And I didn't know, and no one told me.

Dave Souza and his wife Linda agree that prednisone can have some odd psychological effects:

Dave: I was happy when I was taking megadoses of it. I was almost back into the 1960s.

Linda: He was very euphoric right after the surgery, and it continued for a good two weeks when he was home, to the point where he was getting up and fixing me breakfast at five in the morning. He had all this energy. But then, when he fell, boy, it was a hard drop.

Dave: From my point of view, it just intensifies whatever you're feeling.

Linda: In fact, just to show you, he was going to the clinics weekly, every Monday. And there's one pill you're not supposed to take before you go to the clinic.

Dave: They don't want you to take the Neoral the day of your blood test. You take it right after your blood test.

Linda: So, the second clinic date he accidentally took it. And he literally went berserk. He started crying, and oh my God, he just was a mess.

Dave: It's like things become too important. For example, the window-installer just made a nick on our counter, and I was ready to fill the cracks with his flesh. But I'm not violent by nature.

Irritability, restlessness, mood swings, and depression are very common side effects of prednisone, as Jim Gleason discovered:

While my own reactions have been fairly mild and few, they do include the weight gain and mood swings. Mood swings in this case mean something different than what I had expected. Flying off the handle and being upset by things that I would normally have been very patient with in the past is typical. A feeling that everyone else is trying to run my life has turned out to be a form of paranoia associated with the medications, one that has diminished as they have lowered the dosage and allowing me to see that it is me at the root of the feeling, not the actual events around me or others doing it to me.

My patient wife even was driven to call the hospital transplant team and ask, "Who is this monster you sent home to us?" (This is funny in retrospect, but it sure wasn't to her at the time.) They explained that it's just like a woman going through PMS, and to hang in there as it should get better in three months or so. Her patience (and that of the whole family) has been truly tested, but she passed, even when I didn't. Hopefully that is fast becoming a thing of the past as the steroids are lowered and our understanding increases.

Melanie Horne has found the side effects from prednisone to be particularly disturbing:

Prednisone is a nasty drug. Everyone I know [who takes it] has a side effect of the prednisone they don't like. Myself, I have a lot of restlessness, a lot of problems with sleep. We had gotten me down to 10 mg every other day, and that had made a great difference, but since the rejection episode last year they bumped me back up to 10 mg every day. Now I get a lot of nightmares, blood and guts nightmares, really scary stuff, panic, claustrophobia. I've never had any of these kind of things before. I wake up screaming sometimes. Everything seems exaggerated. I also get very, very frightened out on the streets. Without my service dog, I'd be too scared to go out. When somebody does something stupid while driving, there's this big overwhelming feeling, "Oh my God, every car within 100 yards is going to go crunch and I'm going to be in the middle of it." That has got to be the worst side effect of the stuff. I've had a really tough time with it.

I was talking with my pharmacist yesterday, because occasionally I'll get this sensation that's very similar to cramming for finals, as if it's three o'clock in the morning, you've been through three packs of cigarettes and about ten pots of coffee, and you're hoping to God you don't fail the test. And that's the feeling, that sort of mental exhaustion and a little coffee jitter sort of thing. She seems to think that's from prednisone also.

If your psychological side effects from prednisone are extremely severe, your doctor may prescribe anti-psychotic medications to relieve them. Severe reactions are very unusual. Much more common are mild reactions such as the aforementioned euphoria and irritability. And when your doctor begins lowering your dose of prednisone you may begin to feel depression.

An excellent resource for people experiencing the physical and psychological side effects of prednisone is the book *Coping with Prednisone*, which was written by two sisters. When Eugenia Zukerman was taking high doses of prednisone for a lung disorder, her sister, Julie R. Inglefinger, MD, helped her understand and deal with its effects.

In addition to suggesting recipes and exercises that help keep the weight gain down, the authors provide several suggestions for dealing with prednisone's psychological effects. They suggest that you expect the mood swings and try to remember that they are temporary and related to an important part of your therapy. They recommend calming yourself with positive affirmations and stress-reduction techniques. They suggest that you make your family and friends aware of this effect of your medication. If you find the psychological effects especially disabling you should ask for a referral to a psychiatrist or a psychopharmacologist, who may be able to control your symptoms with other medications.

Another informative prednisone resource was written by Jeffrey D. Punch, MD, a transplant surgeon at the University of Michigan Medical Center. His article "Your Child and Prednisone," is available online at *http://www.classkids.org/library/pred.htm*.

Cyclosporine

Cyclosporine is probably the second most common drug taken by transplant patients. Cyclosporine is the generic name for this drug, which is also known as Cyclosporin A or CsA. Cyclosporine has two trade-name formulations: Neoral and Sandimmune, both made by Novartis (formerly Sandoz) Pharmaceuticals. There is also a newly available generic version, which is sold at a much lower price, but Novartis is challenging the U.S. Food and Drug Administration's approval of the generic form, claiming that it is not truly equivalent to the trade-name versions.

The introduction of cyclosporine in the early 1980s was directly responsible for the increased success of organ transplantation. Together with prednisone, it very effectively suppresses the body's rejection of the new organ.

Although its mode of action is poorly understood, cyclosporine seems to interfere with the T cells of the immune system.

Cyclosporine formulations

Both Neoral and Sandimmune are available in injectable forms for use in the hospital, but once you get home you'll be taking them as a liquid or in soft gelatin capsules. If you take the liquid form, you'll measure out your prescribed dose using a measuring syringe. Place the liquid into a glass or ceramic mug and mix it thoroughly with room-temperature orange or apple juice. Milk makes cyclosporine taste unpleasant, and you should never take it with grapefruit or grapefruit juice, which can affect cyclosporine metabolism. Oddly enough, scientists have discovered only in the last few years that there's a substance in grapefruit that affects the cells in your intestine in such a way as to increase the absorption of many different medications.

Many people find gelatin capsules of Neoral or Sandimmune more convenient than the liquid version. Capsules come in both 25 mg and 100 mg versions. The 100 mg capsules are quite large, however, and some people may have difficulty swallowing them.

You may take cyclosporine with or without food, but it's best to take it on the same dosing schedule each day regarding time and meals. This will tend to keep a constant level of the drug in your bloodstream. The manufacturer also recommends that you store the capsules in the original packaging until at most seven days before use. Some transplant recipients like to distribute a month's worth of pills into one of those handy pill boxes with a compartment for each day. If you do this, distribute only a week's worth of cyclosporine at a time.

It will take your doctor a while to find the proper dose of cyclosporine for you. Everyone metabolizes cyclosporine a bit differently, and especially at the beginning your doctor will have your blood tested for cyclosporine levels frequently to make sure you're receiving a dose that's high enough, but not too high. On days that you're scheduled for a cyclosporine blood test you should not take your regular dose until after your blood has been drawn.

It's important to remember that even though Neoral and Sandimmune are both cyclosporine, they are not exactly equivalent. Cyclosporine alone is a white powder that dissolves very poorly in water. Both Neoral and Sandimmune are suspensions of cyclosporine in oil, but they are formulated differently. Neoral, the newer form, forms a microemulsion that's somewhat easier for your body to absorb. For that reason, if you take 100 mg of Neoral you'll end up with a higher blood level of cyclosporine than if you take 100 mg of Sandimmune. Do not let a pharmacist or a hospital substitute Neoral for Sandimmune, or vice versa, without discussing the change with your doctor.

Side effects

Like prednisone, cyclosporine carries the risk of a number of serious side effects. Probably the most significant is "nephrotoxicity"—it can cause kidney damage. For that reason, if you're taking cyclosporine your doctor will be watching your creatinine levels closely. Creatinine is a substance that's normally excreted by the kidneys. If your blood levels of creatinine are elevated, it's an indication that your kidneys are not doing their job. Elevated creatinine is also an indication that a transplanted kidney may be failing, so if you've had a kidney transplant, it takes an expert eye to differentiate between nephrotoxicity caused by cyclosporine and a rejection episode.

This difficulty in diagnosis is exactly what happened to Lori Noyes two years after her kidney transplant:

> I did have one setback. My creatinine was increasing, and I pointed it out to my doctor. He said, "Your drug levels are fine. Let's just watch it." It was going up a little bit more, and I was getting shakiness in my hands, so I said, "Are you sure my drug levels are okay?" He said, "Everything's fine." Well, by February things weren't fine, and I wasn't feeling well. I was feeling very puffy, and I had this sense of dread. I said to my doctor, "Something is very wrong. I'm swelling up again in my ankles. If I didn't know better I'd say I was in kidney failure again." He could tell I was almost in a panic because I thought I was rejecting. It had been almost two years.

> He looked at the blood test and said, "Your creatinine is 2.7. I think you need a biopsy." I got the biopsy a couple weeks later, and that was the worst time in my life, because I thought I was losing my organ. It turned out that I had toxicity of the kidney from the cyclosporine. So the good news is it wasn't rejection, but the bad news is it was permanent damage, scarring to the kidney, so my creatinine will always be a little abnormal. I didn't have to be in the hospital. It is just a matter of watching the

medications. It was a scare for both of us. I remember my doctor saying, "You know you're my star patient. This can't happen to you." But once they adjusted the medication I felt fine again.

Because of the potential for nephrotoxicity, kidney transplant patients may not be given cyclosporine immediately after transplant. Dr. Randall E. Morris, an expert in anti-rejection medications at Stanford University, explains:

> *In a kidney transplant patient who has had a long period of preservation of kidneys [i.e., a long time between when the organ was retrieved and when it was transplanted], it may take a while for his kidneys to perform normally after reperfusion of blood. He may be on dialysis for a while. So to avoid any insult or injury some people withhold cyclosporine for a few weeks or days until the kidney starts producing urine normally.*

Two other significant side effects of cyclosporine are elevated blood pressure and elevated cholesterol. Your doctor may well prescribe blood pressure medications, such as Minipress or Procardia, and cholesterol lowering medications, such as Pravacol, to alleviate these side effects. Dave Souza explains:

> *Neoral increases my blood pressure at the dosage I'm taking. So I had to increase my Minipress, which makes me very tired and lethargic. When I first started taking it, while I was on dialysis, I had to go to the bathroom in the middle of the night, and I couldn't get to the bathroom, I was that groggy. Now I'm kind of used to it. Another side effect of the Neoral is increases in cholesterol. I've never had a cholesterol problem. I always was around 170 to 180. Well, the last cholesterol test I had I was 267, although they weren't concerned because it hadn't been six months yet. It's another trade-off.*

Gum hyperplasia is another side effect of cyclosporin. Kathryn Flynn describes this unpleasant symptom:

> *I have gum hyperplasia. All of a sudden your gums start growing on top of each other. Mine is not real bad, but apparently it can start to cover your teeth, so it makes it harder to clean your teeth. It's not uncomfortable, it's just kind of yucky-looking. You have to be careful to keep brushing your teeth and flossing really well. I didn't realize how bad it could get, but I just read on the TRNSPLNT mailing list that someone actually had to have those gums cut away, which sounds awful to me.*

Gum hyperplasia can be especially bad in children. Some children need have to have a procedure called a gingivectomy every year or two to have the overgrowth cut away.

Compared to prednisone, cyclosporine causes few psychological reactions, but some patients do experience some confusion, especially at higher doses.

Nephrotoxicity, increases in blood pressure and cholesterol, confusion, and gum hyperplasia are all significant medical consequences of cyclosporine use. A somewhat less significant one is a slight tremor in the hands. But the side effect of cyclosporine that creates the most discussion among transplant recipients is probably the least significant medically: it causes abnormal hair growth, also known as hirsutism. As Dave Souza explains, this isn't much of a problem for most men:

> My barber loves it. He wants me to give it to all his customers. I shave my ears now, which I'm not proud of. I look like [actor] Robin Williams under my clothes, although I don't have his salary. My bald spot disappeared for a while, but it'll come back.

Women, on the other hand, tend to worry much more about abnormal hair growth. Melanie Horne points out that not all of this hair growth is bad:

> Your hair grows like mad. I remember a discussion on the TRNS-PLNT email list that must have gone on for three months with people talking about how to get rid of hair. Some people who were losing their hair before transplant now have had it grow back. I've got this incredibly long, huge ponytail. I stopped trying to cut it because I'd just have to go back for another haircut in another two or three weeks.

But Lori Noyes noticed excessive "peach fuzz":

> The good hair growth was on my head, because my hair was thinning and almost gone with the kidney failure and the diabetes. I have nice long hair now. It also grows on my lower back. It bothers me that I have extra hair there, like peach fuzz. On my face—I'm a fair-haired person, blonde basically, so it doesn't show, and I don't have to shave my cheeks or anything, but it's definitely peach fuzz. Above my lips I do shave because it gets dark there. I also think it grows in a little more coarsely and vigorously on my legs. I don't get it sprouting out of my chest or anything weird. It was four months before this happened. I've seen transplant patients walk out of the hospital looking like apes, so I am luckier than others.

Here are some suggestions for dealing with the excess hair from cyclosporine:

- Waxing is effective, but painful. Some recipients recommend a product called Sugar Wax.

- Depilatories are over-the-counter liquids or creams, such as Nair or Surgi-Cream, that dissolve and remove hair. Some people find them quite effective, and Kathryn Flynn says, "I keep the wax company and the Nair company in business."

- Bleaching can be effective for small quantities of hair, but Jim Gleason quotes a woman who recalls that when she tried to bleach her jet black eyebrows, they ended up looking like the fur of a calico cat.

- Shaving is a basic option, although many women don't like to shave their faces, because the hair seems to grow back thicker.

- Electric hair trimmers can be especially effective for excess arm hair.

- Electrolysis and laser hair removal are often not as permanent as their practitioners would have you believe. Also, these techniques can be quite expensive.

- A professional hairstylist may be able to trim your eyebrows to make them look thinner, and can dye them to match your hair.

- Tweezing is not recommended, because it can lead to infections that can become quite serious in an immunosuppressed person.

Prograf (tacrolimus)

Prograf is the trade name of a relatively new immunosuppressant known generically as tacrolimus, and it's manufactured by Fujisawa. While it was in clinical trials it was also known by the code name FK506, and many physicians are still in the habit of referring to it by that designation.

Prograf seems to work in a way very similar to cyclosporine in inhibiting the immune system's T cells. While it has a similar pattern of nephrotoxicity, it does not promote gum thickening or abnormal hair growth. For that reason, Prograf may be a particularly good option for some women.

Prograf is not without side effects, however. Among the potential adverse reactions listed are headache, tremor, hair loss, diarrhea, nausea, muscle cramps, vomiting, irregular heartbeat, high blood pressure, and increases in blood sugar.

Prograf has some fairly common psychological side effects as well, including abnormal dreams, agitation, anxiety, confusion, convulsions (seizures), hallucinations, mental depression, and nervousness.

Dr. Morris describes how some transplant physicians use Prograf:

> It's a harder drug than cyclosporine to learn how to use. But now with more experience more and more physicians are using it. It's often used now for people who are on Neoral who have one rejection episode after the other. We might switch from Neoral to Prograf.

You should take Prograf one hour before or two hours after meals. Like cyclosporine, you should not take Prograf with grapefruit or grapefruit juice. Absorption of Prograf can change if you change the type or the amount of food you eat. Consult with your doctor before changing your diet. And it's important to maintain a very regular dosing schedule to keep your blood levels constant. Usually you'll be told to take a dose every twelve hours. If you miss a dose, and you realize this within a few hours, take the missed dose as soon as you remember. But if it's almost time for your next dose, skip the missed dose, go back to your regular schedule, and check with your doctor. Do not take a double dose if you miss a dose.

Imuran (azathioprine)

Imuran is the trade name of a drug called azathioprine, which has been used in transplant patients for about 40 years. It's manufactured by the Burroughs Wellcome Co. It seems to work by inhibiting cell division.

Imuran can cause some serious side effects. One of the most serious is that it can affect your bone marrow, causing significant decreases in white blood cells, which fight infection, and platelets, which help your blood clot. You should contact your doctor immediately if you notice unusual bleeding or bruising. On the other hand, you should not stop taking Imuran unless your doctor tells you to. You should also call your doctor immediately if you feel any unusual tiredness or weakness.

Other significant side effects include nausea, vomiting, and diarrhea. You may be able to lessen this effect by taking your Imuran after meals or at bedtime. Imuran can also cause fever, chills, and skin rash.

If you have gout and are being treated with allopurinal (Zyloprim), you should know that Imuran interacts with this medication to increase damage to your bone marrow. If you're on Imuran and a doctor prescribes allopurinol (or vice versa) make sure she knows about your other medications.

If you miss a dose of Imuran, your response will depend on whether you're taking it several times a day or only once. If you're taking several doses a day and you miss one, doctors generally recommend doubling up on the next dose. But if you're taking only a single dose a day, do not take the missed dose at all and do not double the next one. Instead, go back to your regular dosing schedule and check with your doctor.

CellCept (mycophenolate mofetil)

CellCept is the trade name of a fairly new drug called mycophenolate mofetil, which was developed by Roche Pharmaceuticals. It seems to work by interfering with the immune system's T cells and B cells.

Side effects of CellCept seem relatively mild compared to some other immunosuppressants. CellCept can cause neutropenia, which is a significant lowering in the number of white blood cells. If you're on CellCept, your white blood cell count will be monitored closely. Other potential side effects include diarrhea, vomiting, and the risk of serious blood infections.

Dr. Dafoe explains the tradeoffs between CellCept and cyclosporine:

> Cyclosporine can cause kidney dysfunction, but it's just such a good drug, and the nephrotoxicity is reversible. It's related to the blood level, so it's a matter of dosing appropriately. Also there's something called chronic cyclosporine toxicity, but over time we've added CellCept, which is a good drug that has allowed us to lower the cyclosporine levels and therefore avoid some of the nephrotoxicity.

Rapamune (sirolimus)

Late in 1999, the US Food and Drug Administration (FDA) approved a new drug called Rapamune (sirolimus is the generic name) to fight organ rejection in kidney recipients. Manufactured by Wyeth-Ayerst, a division of American Home Products, Rapamune seems to work by preventing the proliferation of T cells. The major advantage of Rapamune is that it is less likely to damage the kidney than is cyclosporine. Rapamune does have some known side effects of its own—it increases cholesterol levels, for example—but its full side-effect profile won't be known until physicians have the experience of prescribing it to large numbers of kidney recipients.

Other medications

Because anti-rejection drugs tend to cause so many side effects, you will likely be taking some medications intended to control those side effects. We'll briefly mention some of those medications here. For further information, ask your doctor or pharmacist, or consult one of the many good drug references available in bookstores. On the Internet, the Mayo Clinic maintains an excellent site were you can look up detailed information on more than 8,000 prescription drugs. You'll find the Mayo Clinic Medicine Center at *http://mayohealth.org/usp/common/index.htm.*

Because you're immunosuppressed, you're much more likely to catch bacterial or viral infections. For that reason your doctor may well prescribe an antibiotic and/or an antiviral for you to take regularly to prevent infection. Frequently Bactrim (sulfamethoxazole) will be the antibiotic, and Zovirax (acyclovir) will be the antiviral.

If you're having nephrotoxicity or some other kidney problems, you may be retaining water. If so, your doctor may prescribe Lasix (furosemide), a diuretic.

Both cyclosporine and prednisone can cause elevated cholesterol. In addition to asking you to modify your diet, your doctor may prescribe Lipitor (atorvastatin) or Pravachol (pravastatin) to help lower your cholesterol.

Cyclosporine and prednisone can both also cause elevated blood pressure. There is a large number of medications your doctor can prescribe to lower your blood pressure, including Procardia (nifedipine), Tenormin (atenolol), and Vasotec (enalapril)

Some immunosuppressants cause stomach upset. There is a variety of medications your doctor may prescribe for this, including Pepcid (famotidine), Zantac (ranitidine), and Prilosec (omeprazole).

Detecting rejection

The first step in dealing with a rejection episode is detecting it. In the early days of transplants, the first sign of rejection in people with kidney transplants might be some tenderness around the new kidney. But these days, no matter what kind of transplant you have, your doctor is likely to detect the first signs of rejection before you notice a thing.

It's sometimes difficult to detect rejection, even for specialists. Sometimes the symptoms of infection can seem very similar to those of rejection. Of course it's critical to determine which is which, since if you're having an infection the treatment may involve backing off on the immunosuppressive medications, while, on the contrary, if you're having a rejection episode the treatment usually involves giving high doses of immunosuppressives.

If you've had a heart transplant, you'll be asked to come in periodically for routine heart biopsies. These sound much worse than they really are. They're usually performed weekly for the first month or so after transplant, and then every other week for two more months. With no evidence of rejection, the frequency of biopsy is reduced to once every two or three months. Different transplant teams have different preferences in these matters, and the frequency may also depend on whether there have been other suspicious signs.

Heart biopsies take only a few minutes, and are normally conducted on an outpatient basis. Under local anesthesia, a device called a bioptome is inserted into a large vein, usually the jugular vein on the right side of your neck. A bioptome is a long, flexible tube that's snaked through your circulatory system until it reaches the right ventricle of your heart. Within the bioptome is a small pair of pincers that grabs three to six tiny pieces of tissue. This tissue is sent to the pathology lab for analysis. The pathologist looks to see how many lymphocytes—white blood cells—are mixed in with the heart muscle cells. Too many and you may be having a rejection episode.

Heart-transplant recipient Jim Gleason wrote this soon after his first (and so far only) rejection episode:

> With each passing biweekly biopsy without signs of rejection, those steroids get reduced to see if they can still balance between rejection and infection. This past week, at exactly the three-month milestone, rejection was found! The body's white cells were able to become too active after the most recent steroid reduction and started to attack the "foreign" heart. Somehow I can picture the red cells saying: "Hey! That's not our heart— you white cells, go get it! Attack! Protect!!" Meanwhile I'm up here looking in telling them all: "Hey guys, that's a friend keeping us all alive! Make peace, not war!"
>
> Things happened fast. The transplant team had educated us well and we knew to expect such rejection—it's a normal part of the process, but still not wanted, of course. . . . You treat rejection before the patient even

knows of any symptoms by the at-home infusion of an increased steroid dosage—fifty times greater than the normal daily dosage!—but only for three days. . . . Within twenty minutes of being notified of the rejection, the home care pharmacy was scheduling delivery of an IV pole and three bags of medicine and associated needles. . . . I continue to feel great, but then the transplant team always said they would know I was in trouble long before I would ever know of it.

If you've had a kidney, pancreas, or liver transplant, you will have far less frequent biopsies. That's because analysis of your blood work shows other early warning signs of rejection—increased creatinine for the kidney patient, increased blood sugar for the pancreas patient, and abnormal liver enzymes for the liver patient. There's no equivalent blood test that indicates the rejection of a heart. Occasionally, especially in the kidney transplant patient, your doctor may ask you to undergo an ultrasound exam if he suspects rejection.

Dr. Dafoe describes how physicians go about detecting rejection in kidney and pancreas patients:

More and more, detecting rejection is a matter of blood work. The symptoms of rejection [in the kidney patient] are fever, malaise, high blood pressure, decreased urine output, and tenderness around the kidney. But because the drugs are so good now, the symptoms have become more and more subtle and it's mainly a change in the creatinine in the blood work. For a pancreas the main sign of rejection is when blood sugar levels, which have been under good control, begin to go up.

Occasionally we still lose a graft due to rejection, but it's become unusual. Nowadays only about 30 percent of kidney recipients have a single rejection episode. So that means a great majority never have a rejection, which is just astoundingly different than the old days. For kidney-pancreas recipients the incidence of rejection is higher, probably more like 50 to 60 percent.

If it looks as if someone is having a rejection episode, we try to rule out other things, because we don't want to immunosuppress if they've got something else going on like an infection. So there's a very definite algorithm that we follow. If someone comes in with their creatinine up, for example, we'll ask, "Are they dehydrated? Are they on any new meds?" and so on.

> *If they are having a rejection episode, we'll usually give them high-dose steroids by IV. If that fails, then they get an anti-T-cell preparation, either a monoclonal antibody or a heterologous anti-lymphocyte antibody. Usually we can tell after three days of steroid treatment whether they're going to need something more. Sometimes it's so bad we go right to the big guns.*

Of course, doctors are not perfect. Melanie Horne, a kidney-pancreas recipient, encountered an inexperienced or inattentive physician who reacted too slowly to the early signs of rejection. She believes that if she had been more aggressive in demanding an immediate biopsy, the outcome may have been different. (While we won't mention the name of the doctor or the hospital here, please note that none of the hospitals, transplant teams, or physicians mentioned in this book were in any way involved in the following incident.)

> *After a clinic visit, they sent me home with a very drastic change in my cyclosporine dosage. And I questioned it again and again. I said, "This is kind of drastic. Are you sure?" They insisted that my lab values indicated that there were toxic levels of cyclosporine in my blood. Basically I was told, "Don't be a pain. Do what you're told and change your medication." Six weeks later I came back with the symptoms of acute rejection due to sub-therapeutic levels of immunosuppressive drugs. When I came in, the transplant surgeon insisted that at five-and-a-half years out from transplant there was no possible way that I was in acute rejection. But it was pointed out to him that my cyclosporine level was a third of what it should have been. Even with that piece of information he refused to do a biopsy right then. Instead he sent me home, and scheduled me for an elective biopsy, but of course by then it was too late, the pancreas was already gone.*

> *I was especially offended when I came in with acute rejection and the transplant surgeon said, "Parts wear out. I don't care." That's a direct quote. He meant, "You're getting older, your pancreas is wearing out and I don't care about it," as if I should just accept it, it's just wearing out. The reality was, I was in acute rejection, and there was something they could have done if they had interjected then, and put me on OKT3 or one of those nasty little drugs that turn around rejections. It could have saved it.*

This story does have a happy ending, though. After waiting on the list a second time, Melanie recently received another successful pancreas transplant.

Treating rejection

Once your doctor detects rejection, you can expect to see a rapid and aggressive medical response. Most rejection episodes are treated in the hospital, but if your doctor decides that you only need high-dose steroids, they can occasionally be administered via IV at home.

Frequently, though, your doctor will want to administer one of those "nasty little drugs" that Melanie refers to above. These are extremely powerful medications with serious side effects, but they can truly be lifesavers in the case of a rejection episode. Sometimes they are given as part of the standard therapy immediately after transplant, even if there's no evidence of rejection. Other times they're given only if high doses of steroids don't stop the rejection episode. Still other times they're given whenever there's a rejection episode. Like so many things in transplant medicine, it depends on the style, experiences, and preferences of your transplant team. If your doctor wants you to have this therapy, you will be admitted to the hospital for two weeks or more, so you can be under close medical supervision.

These drugs are all made up of antibodies, and there are two types: polyclonal antibodies and monoclonal antibodies. All of them are designed to interfere with the T cells of the immune system, which are directly responsible for rejection.

The first to be developed were the polyclonal antibodies. If you inject human T cells into rabbits, horses, or other animals, they will produce antibodies against them. If you then draw blood from these animals and isolate the antibodies, you will end up with a mixture of many antibodies against many different substances, including human T cells. If you inject that antibody preparation into a transplant recipient, it will temporarily interfere with all the T cells that might be mounting a rejection response. These medications go by several names, including anti-thymocyte globulin (ATG or Atgam), anti-lymphocyte serum (ALS), and anti-lymphocyte globulin (ALG).

More recently a monoclonal antibody, whose trade name is Orthoclone OKT3, and whose generic name is Muromonab-CD3, has been developed. To make a monoclonal antibody, human T cells are first injected into a mouse. Then the individual mouse cell making the individual anti-T-cell antibody is isolated. That cell is fused to a cancer cell, which gives it the ability to divide forever in the laboratory, all the while producing the antibody. Another type of monoclonal antibody is targeted against a specific protein, called the interleukin-2 receptor, that resides on the surface of acti-vated T cells. This is called the anti-interleukin-2-receptor antibody, or more simply, anti-IL2R.

The advantage of a monoclonal antibody like OKT3 compared to a poly-clonal antibody is that it can be given in much lower quantities, since it con-tains just the single antibody against T cells. Polyclonal antibodies have to be given in such large volumes that a surgical connection to an artery or large vein is sometimes needed. On the other hand, the main disadvantage of OKT3 is that the patient's body tends to synthesize antibodies to the anti-bodies, and these can block OKT3's action. Since there are so many different antibodies in a polyclonal antibody preparation, there's little chance that your antibodies will target the specific ones attacking your T cells.

Interfering with your T cells, as both monoclonal and polyclonal antibodies are intended to do, is a serious business. The T cells release chemicals that cause some very unpleasant reactions, including chest pain, dizziness, fever and chills, wheezing or shortness of breath, headaches, stomach upset, and diarrhea. When you're under medical supervision most of these reactions, while unpleasant, are temporary and are not truly dangerous, and your doc-tor can often prescribe medications that can relieve the discomfort. How-ever, some people can have an allergic reaction to the antibodies, and this can cause anaphylactic shock, a true medical emergency. If you have chest pain, rapid or irregular heartbeat, shortness of breath or wheezing, or swell-ing of the face or throat, check with your doctor or nurse immediately.

Lori Noyes describes her experience with OKT3:

> After my transplant I was given a very strong drug called OKT3. It's given in some centers just prophylactically to prevent a rejection, but it's frequently given if you have an acute rejection episode. They gave this to me as a standard protocol. When they gave it to me the nurse said, "We're going to give you some Tylenol and Benadryl." I said, "So I could have anaphylactic reaction to this?" She said, "Some patients do. You should be fine." I said, "Great." She gave it to me and sure enough within thirty minutes I was going berserk. I had ants in my pants. I had to move. I had to get out of the bed. I told her to remake the bed, that it was too wrin-kled. I knew I was giving her a hard time, but I was feeling out of control, and she never bothered to tell me it was a very common reaction to the OKT3. I had to have fourteen days of this, but luckily I only got that reac-tion the first two days, and then everything was fine.

A patient's philosophy

If you're waiting for or considering a transplant, this chapter may have seemed pretty daunting to you. You've learned about rejection and the long list of medications you'll be taking to stave off rejection, and another set of pills you may be taking to deal with the side effects of the first set. If this seems a bit overwhelming, consider this charming meditation on medication, which Jim Gleason contributed to the TRNSPLNT mailing list not long ago:

> Each week I stand in the kitchen and refill my fourteen-slot pill case—seven mornings, seven evenings worth of life-saving medications. It's been four-and-a-half years now of this weekly ritual. In the early weeks and months it was a daunting task, with a lot of concerns for "quality control"—I would count out each day's ten different pill types by their correct quantities/colors/shapes, while Jay, my wife, would cross-check my accuracy, my hands, shaky from the prednisone, often sending some colored beads flying over the floor (usually under the stove or refrig, out of reach—how frustrating. . .).
>
> As the weeks and months passed, the number of types and quantities of each were tapered down, even to the point where prednisone was no longer part of the daily cocktail mix (after just six months!). Today we live on the basic mix of Neoral and Imuran with some blood pressure and cholesterol control types offsetting their side effects. Yes, a multi-vitamin and some magnesium (to help with the memory, if I recall correctly) round out the daily regimen, and with very few exceptions, the discipline has been very complete with only two forgets over those 1,562 days—not bad, given life's complexity and busyness over these wonderful months since the heart transplant back in October of 1994.

Jim continues, reflecting on his pill ritual:

> Today's ritual is more routine, with quality control solely in my hands. As I stand there and open the week's supply and carefully put each day's mix in the AM and PM slots of the pill case I find myself reflecting on how quickly time passes. Each week seems to come faster than the last, and the pill case is empty yet again. It is an interesting way to measure one's life—counting the weeks like this. You must take this short "time-out" of life to re-supply and I wonder where that week went—again?

Most people I know never stop to think about that passage of time, certainly not on a weekly basis as we do. Another of our "gifts"—this moment to pause and reflect.

So what have we done with the gift of this week of life? Often not a comfortable question to face, the time having come and gone so quickly, it seems, yet another week has passed—the seven days of fourteen empty slots on the counter in front of me attest to that fact. Whom have I touched this past week? How have I shared this gift of "re-birth" with those around me? What lessons have I learned from this week's experiences? How have I communicated to my family how special they have been to be with this past week? Have I gone past the daily "clean the house" and "went to work" to make the days special in some way that will last beyond the daily routine of life? That daily routine is not bad—in fact it is much appreciated now that we who have experienced an organ transplant have seen what life can be without the normal routine that was impossible pre-transplant—returning to routine is something we now live to celebrate, but today, post-transplant, there is so much more.

Looking ahead at his life, Jim measures it out in weekly doses:

I pop the Neoral packages—three of the 25 mg capsules and one of the 100s for the morning, and again for the evening dose—and amidst the wonder of its miracle and dangers the slots get filled, one by one, as I look up and think ahead to the days of the coming week when these meds will be taken. What will I do with this week? What meetings—both business and volunteer/support group—will I attend and how will I contribute to those meetings? What special thing can we do as a family this week—making sure to insert into the business work week special moments of family time and celebration. No longer will the days be taken for granted, after all, that's what these pills serve as a reminder of. Those days almost didn't come for us—for me—and most importantly, some day they will run out, and pills will be left over in those daily slots, unfinished. But until then, the challenge of this week—this gift of time—weighs on my mind... and each week that challenge is different—the opportunity changing—an opportunity that can be taken advantage of or missed—that is my choice.

The last pill is put into its slot—mixing with the colors and shapes of the others that have gone before it—a note is made to order a refill for the

*near empty bottle of one or another, in time to avoid the panic of the
totally empty container (no easy task, what with doctor prescriptions that
need to be rewritten regularly, and mail-order pharmacies that delay, or
deliveries that are not left for lack of signatures, etc.). The big plastic hon-
eycombed pill box is replaced up in the kitchen cabinet to await its daily
life-saving ritual. So problematic, yet so relatively simple when one stops
to think of its place in this total transplant experience. Yes, amazing! And
another week of seven days, pills taken twice a day, fourteen times before
it is time to repeat this pause for reflection on the fleeting nature of life,
a time passage totally independent of the transplant, yet we are gifted
with this ritual opportunity to take time to stop and reflect—as we refill
those pill slots—hopefully for many, many years to come. . . .*

So what have you done with this week just past?

*And, more importantly, what are you going to do with your week,
this week, before the seven days have past and it is time to ask those questions yet again?*

*As for me, I shared and expressed my love with several very special
people, re-filled my pill box, and, of course, wrote this piece of sharing
and challenge for you.*

Jim's meditation makes the point that you shouldn't go through the enormous hassle of a transplant and its aftermath merely to stay alive. You should
do it in order to live a full life. How to do that is the subject of the next
chapter.

CHAPTER 9

Living with a Transplant

MANY MEDICAL PROFESSIONALS like to remind patients that when you get a transplant, you're not simply curing your illness. Instead, you're trading one medical condition for another. Before the transplant you may have had heart disease, kidney disease, or liver disease, but afterward you have to deal with the significant effects of being immunosuppressed. As you will see in this chapter, dealing with your post-transplant medical condition is much more complicated than merely remembering to take all your medications on time.

Kidney-pancreas recipient Melanie Horne describes the importance of taking control of your life:

> I think it's really important to take full responsibility for your well-being. A transplant is not something that's just done and over with. You've got to be committed to it. You've got to take control of everything that affects your life. If there are problems, fix them. Figure out a way. I think the patients who expect it to be just taken care of behind their backs and just don't want to hear about it probably won't do as well as those who are willing to be committed to educating themselves and taking responsibility.

On the other hand, a happy post-transplant life involves much more than just worrying about your medical condition. The enormous hassle of major surgery and its aftermath would hardly be worth it unless the transplant allowed you to live a life full of everything life has to offer. While years of declining health and anxiety about your medical condition may conspire to keep you from a full post-transplant life, most transplant recipients can and should live life to the fullest.

In this chapter, we'll look first at a number of issues on the subject of managing your medication. We'll discuss how to keep your drugs straight, how to identify yourself with a medical ID, how to receive proper treatment in an emergency or at a strange hospital, and how to think about over-the-counter and herbal medications. We'll then look at how to keep from getting infections while immunosuppressed. Next, we'll give some necessary warnings about cancer and cancer screening. We'll close with a look at the fun stuff: living life with gusto.

Dealing with your medication

Chapter 8, *Anti-Rejection Drugs*, looks at some of the medications that you as a transplant patient are likely to be taking. It takes a while to get used to the complex regimen of your medications, especially in the weeks immediately after transplant.

During that period you'll be taking an especially large number of drugs, and your doctor may be adjusting the dosages frequently. You'll be taking some of the pills once a day, some twice, and some more frequently. You'll be taking some with meals, and some at least an hour or two before or after meals.

After several weeks or months, things should get a bit easier. Your dosages will decline and then stabilize, and you may be able to get off some medications entirely.

Heart-transplant recipient Jim Gleason has some very practical and down-to-earth advice regarding drugs. To begin with, to help you keep your medications straight, you should maintain an up-to-date list of all of them, he recommends:

> My medicine regimen is very complex. I found it useful to maintain (on my personal computer) a record of what prescriptions I was taking, including the generic names, dosage levels, scheduled times for taking them, and finally a brief note as to what they were for. This came in handy in many ways, and I strongly recommend you come up with your own way of doing this same thing.

> First, it gave us a place to immediately record the changes that the transplant team called with after biopsies, thus our filling of those daily dosages were done against that form and always current. Second, carrying that same form with your driver's license makes it available for emergency personnel in the case of an accident or emergency. That's where the police look first when they come upon a victim—for identification. The EMT [Emergency Medical Technician] will need to know that you are immune-suppressed, that the typical heart symptoms may be different in a heart transplant patient's case, and what meds you are taking. With so

many prescriptions, don't count on anyone (including yourself, [as you] may be incoherent at the time of the emergency) to be able to relate the full list (and amounts). In some cases, the EMT will not be familiar with some of the special prescriptions we take (hence the need for a couple of words on that form that tell what each medication is for).

In the home, that medication list should be posted on the refrigerator door—again, that's the first place they're trained to look. Whenever I went to the doctor's, the emergency room, or even to the transplant clinic, everyone was delighted to find this information so well organized and complete.

You may also wish to put a bit of information about your medical insurance on this document. It's a good idea to have the name of your plan, your provider, your identification number, the plan's telephone number, and a telephone number for your transplant team with you at all times.

Medical identification

Some transplant teams provide a wallet-sized medical identification card for their patients. While this card will not normally have the level of detail about your exact dosages that Jim's list does, it will advertise the fact that you're a transplant patient on immunosuppressive medications, and it will provide telephone numbers for medical personnel to call for more information.

But it's not enough just to carry this information in your wallet. You may find yourself in a strange city needing medical attention after your wallet has been lost or stolen. In an emergency situation, you may become separated from your wallet. Some agencies have policies prohibiting an EMT from opening your wallet unless a second EMT or a police officer is present. For that reason, you should definitely acquire a bracelet or pendant with your medical information etched into it, and wear it constantly.

While some transplant programs provide their own ID jewelry, and some life insurance companies provide a similar service to their clients, most patients will purchase ID tags from the non-profit MedicAlert Foundation. When you buy a bracelet or pendant from them, you're buying much more than a piece of jewelry. You're buying the services of a 24-hour emergency response center that stores your confidential medical information, including details about your medical condition and your medications—along with their exact dosages.

Only a small amount of information can actually fit on a MedicAlert tag. There's space for about 90 characters on the regular version and 60 characters on the small version. But that's more than enough to print "Kidney Transplant Steroids Immunosuppressants Hypertensive," for example. In addition to those 60 or 90 characters, the ID tag contains your unique member number and a telephone number that medical personnel worldwide are instructed to call collect for more information. The emergency response center can transmit your detailed medical information anywhere in the world, any time of the day, in any of 140 different languages.

The MedicAlert service costs $35 for the first year and $15 for each subsequent year. For that cost, you get a basic stainless steel bracelet. Other styles have a slightly higher initial cost. For example, if your skin reacts badly to stainless steel (some people are allergic to the nickel contained in most stainless-steel alloys), you can get a hypoallergenic, titanium-coated bracelet for $50. Whatever style you choose, you'll be able to change your medical information on file as frequently as you wish.

For more information, contact the MedicAlert Foundation at (800) 432-5378 or online at *http://www.medicalert.org/*.

Over-the-counter medications

You should never take any kind of over-the-counter medicines or herbal remedies without checking with your transplant team first.

Many people have the idea that if you can walk into a drugstore or supermarket and buy a medication without a prescription, that means the government has determined that it's completely safe. This is an entirely erroneous idea, especially for transplant patients. Many over-the-counter medications can cause serious side effects, and worse, they can interact badly with some of the medications you're already taking.

For example, the common analgesic ibuprofen makes the kidneys more sensitive to the toxic effects of cyclosporine. Ibuprofen is sold as a generic and under several trade names, including Motrin and Advil, and it can also be one ingredient among many in sinus remedies and cold medications. This side effect of ibuprofen is shared by other "non-steroidal anti-inflammatory drugs" (NSAIDs), a group that includes aspirin, naproxen sodium, and many others.

Common antacids are another example of a seemingly harmless over-the-counter drug that can interact with the medications you're taking. Antacids can slow down the absorption of your other drugs from your stomach.

Grapefruit and grapefruit juice, on the other hand, have recently been shown to significantly increase the absorption of many drugs from the intestinal tract. This can result in higher than normal blood levels of cyclosporine and other medications.

It's not only certain foods and regular over-the-counter medicines that you have to watch out for. Many people now like to take herbal remedies, thousands of which are sold freely in health-food stores or ethnic pharmacies as pills, capsules, extracts, and teas. While some herbal remedies are harmless, others contain powerful drugs that can interact with your prescribed medication in unpredictable ways. It may surprise you to learn that unlike over-the-counter or prescription medications, no government agency examines the purity, safety, or efficacy of herbal remedies.

When admitted to a hospital

Because of the unique medical needs of transplant patients, transplant teams used to recommend that you visit your original team at your original hospital for any medical problem, even the most minor ones, such as a hangnail. All transplant teams are housed within "tertiary-care" hospitals. These are facilities with the most modern equipment, and they are able to provide the most advanced level of care. Unfortunately, many transplant patients don't live close to their transplant team. Also, your health plan may not allow you to go to your transplant team for routine care. And in emergency situations, you'll likely be taken to whatever hospital is closest.

Stanford cardiologist Sharon A. Hunt, MD, thinks that this can present serious problems:

> We used to try to get patients to come back here with all their medical problems, but it's frankly just not practical anymore. Most of the time, even with serious complications, the HMOs won't let them come back. It's a big problem. We're talking about big medical problems that physicians outside tertiary-care centers don't feel comfortable handling, but they are being forced to handle them because the HMO won't let patients come back to the tertiary-care center.

A clear example happened to us last week. I got a call from a patient's physician, and the patient was clearly developing a malignancy. These patients get very unusual kinds of malignancies, and they really ought to be taken care of at a tertiary-care center that has experience with this. So the doctor and I immediately arranged for the patient to come here the next morning. When he didn't show up, I called to find out why not, and the doctor was just aghast that the HMO wouldn't let the patient come back to Stanford. They told the doctor he had to take care of it. We're still fighting that one, but that's the sort of bind we get into quite a lot at hospitals.

If you find yourself admitted to a hospital away from your transplant team, you will have to be especially vigilant to make sure you're getting proper medical care. You should insist that the doctors consult with members of your transplant team when deciding on treatment. If they won't call, you must. You should also make sure they're giving you the correct medications.

Normally when you're admitted to a hospital you won't be permitted to take your own medications into the room with you. That's because the hospital wants to maintain absolute control over your prescriptions. But this policy can cause problems that you have to keep a close eye on. For example, it can take a long time for the new pharmacy to fill your prescription. If you suspect that you're in danger of missing a dose, you'll have to insist on faster service, or you'll have to insist on taking medicine you brought from home.

You can also find yourself in a worse predicament. Sometimes doctors and pharmacists who are not familiar with immunosuppressive medications will blindly substitute one form of cyclosporine for another. If you're on Neoral and the pharmacy delivers Sandimmune or a generic, you're going to have to demand a switch.

This is definitely not the time to be timid, to be a "good patient." This is the time to be assertive, to be firm, and if necessary, to be a royal pain in the neck.

Lisa G. Levin, a nurse coordinator in Stanford's Department of Cardiothoracic Surgery, emphasizes the need for transplant patients to take charge of their own medical care:

We give them a card to carry that says, "Please contact Stanford. This is a transplant recipient." But the best advocate and the last line of defense is that patient. They have to take responsibility for the fact that they shouldn't just blindly be putting medications into their mouths that they don't know about. We spend a lot of time talking about this because they can get into trouble. The best thing they can do when a local physician is prescribing medication for them, and they are in doubt, is to call us. We can tell them whether it's okay or if there is an alternate drug that would be safer.

Dr. Hunt says that patients should, if necessary, loudly demand quality care:

I think they should be very, very vocal about [quality of treatment]. When doctors complain about these things, it comes across as very self-serving, but if patients start being proactive and loud about the suboptimal care that's being allowed, I think it will have a lot better effect. I'm always encouraging patients to voice their unhappiness about that system. If the patient feels they're getting the wrong medicine at the wrong time, then they have to go to their doctor and say, "Look, this is the way it's got to be."

Avoiding infection

At one point in Homer's epic poem *The Odyssey*, the Greek hero Odysseus has to navigate his ship through a narrow passage in the Straits of Messina. On one side is Scylla, a fearsome sea monster with six heads and twelve feet. On the other is Charybdis, a whirlpool that devours entire ships. Odysseus makes it through, just barely, but his ship and his men are destroyed.

Your transplant team will be navigating you through an equally narrow passage. If they give you lots of immunosuppressants, you'll avoid the Scylla of rejection, but you may pass too close to the Charybdis of infection.

Avoiding the twin perils of rejection and infection requires vigilance, skillful medical care, and close cooperation between you and your transplant team. To guard against infection, your doctor may put you on a steady dose of antibiotics and antiviral medications even when you're not sick. But there are also many other things you can do yourself to ward off infection. Jim Gleason describes his initial worries about infection and how he dealt with them:

It's a scary time, living with a suppressed immune system, especially those first couple of years. With all the warnings, watching for signs and symptoms, answering the regular questions of the doctors and nurses (not to mention the family who alertly monitor your every action for anything different, followed by their loving: "What's the matter?"), it is very easy to wonder if you are getting paranoid. I seldom paid any attention to aches and pains—they would go away over time, I was sure. Now, I was expected to constantly be on the alert, to fill in by observation for the body's immune system that was kept from working by the medications that assured life in this post-transplant world.

This can only be imagined by those around us. Only now do we realize just how amazing this body of ours is, with its automatic protection system no longer taken for granted. A simple sniffle, a runny nose, a sneeze is "nothing to be sneezed at," and the concern level rises fast the first couple of times you face them in this new world. You listen intently at the wheeze. Am I developing pneumonia? This always happens on a Friday evening—or going into a long holiday weekend—when you least expect to be able to reach your transplant doctor. So you err on the side of over-caution, and a friendly nurse calls back with some questions and finally the directive to "take a couple of Tylenol and call us" if this or that happens. Whew, relief! But you still lie there as you enter the night of sleep, and wonder, listening for the sounds deep inside that were so familiar before transplant. They don't come. Sleep does. And you awake to another wonderful day. You do feel foolish, at first, but there are so many stories where fellow patients didn't call and they should have. You get used to it. You get back to living the "normal" life again. As the months pass, the immune system is balanced with the regimen of meds, biopsies testifying to their effectiveness each couple of weeks, then every month, then every three months, and you look forward to the time when these will be done only twice a year.

Suggestions for avoiding infection include taking special care just after transplant, staying away from crowds, avoiding sick people, washing frequently with antibacterial soap, being careful when preparing chicken and other animal products, avoiding shellfish, making sure water is safe, and taking precautions around pets. This list of suggestions may at first seem long, and it may seem impossible that you can obey all of them. But rest assured that they'll become second nature fairly quickly.

The riskiest time is in the weeks and months immediately after transplant, when you'll be on the highest doses of immunosuppressants. You'll be able to let down your guard a bit after a while, as did Steve Rahn:

> During that first six months, the medical staff of course suggested caution. I certainly avoided the kinds of things that would quickly get me in trouble—crowds with people who could have colds, children who had chicken pox or measles, and those kinds of things. I became very conscious of good personal hygiene habits. But I really didn't give it much thought after that. Once the doctors said, "As long as you're feeling well, and as long as you avoid these obvious risk generators, you'll be all right," I took that to heart and really went all out.

As Steve says, you should stay away from crowds at first. This is particularly important during the winter cold and flu season. You don't want to be going to large parties, to shopping malls, to sporting events, and the like. Whenever there are many people gathered together, some will be ill, and they'll be coughing and sneezing, spreading their germs hither and yon.

On the other hand, you shouldn't panic if your wife or kids get a cold. There's no need for you to live in an enclosed bubble. Transplant nurse Lisa G. Levin describes what she tells patients:

> If a recipient's spouse gets the flu soon after transplant, we would probably see if there was an alternate caregiver who could be accessed, not only for the recipient, but for the support person. They need to be able to have their time to recover from illness as well. But later on in the course, generally hand-washing is the best message. Patients should also make sure that tissues are kept separate, and that they're not cleaning up their family member's tissues.
>
> We're not suppressing their immune system so much that viruses would be deadly, but they may just experience a virus a little worse, or have a little bit sicker course than someone else. Ideally, you want to remove whoever is infected, but we have many recipients who are parents, and they have to take care of their kids. For the most part, our belief is that we haven't suppressed them so much that it's lethal for them to have that kind of exposure. The idea after transplant is to live your life, and we don't want everybody so restricted or so paranoid about those types of issues that they're not getting the best quality of life that they can have.

Make sure there's plenty of antibacterial soap in every bathroom and at every kitchen sink in your house. Wash your hands frequently. Carry antibacterial hand wash with you, the kind that doesn't require water, when you go out.

There are many precautions you should take that are related to food. The kitchen can be the most germ-filled part of your house, what with all the food lying around. You should keep counters clean, and dishes washed, using antibacterial cleansers. And you should get rid of old food before it starts turning into science projects in the refrigerator.

Some foods require special preparation. Raw chicken and eggs can harbor salmonella bacteria and should be handled carefully and thoroughly cooked. Wash your hands immediately after touching raw chicken. Beware of handling cooked chicken with the same utensils used for raw chicken. Don't put cooked chicken on the same plate that held it when it was raw. Cook your eggs to firmness. If your whites or yolks are still runny, that's an indication that you haven't gotten them hot enough to kill the bacteria.

Red meat can harbor the E. coli bacteria. Hamburger should be cooked until it's brown inside and out—"medium" at least. If you prefer your meat rare or medium rare, stick to steaks. E. coli can't penetrate far into the interior of a solid piece of meat, so cooking the outside thoroughly is enough. But when you grind steak for hamburger, any E. coli on the outside will be distributed throughout the meat.

Pork can carry trichinosis, and should always be cooked thoroughly. Never eat rare pork.

You should avoid all shellfish, especially raw clams or oysters. Many perfectly healthy people with intact immune systems are sickened by shellfish every year, and the risk is much greater if you're immunocompromised. Sushi and sashimi—raw fish dishes served at Japanese restaurants—should also be avoided.

Being aware of such things is not that difficult, even when you're away from home, explains Steve Rahn:

> I'm really conscious about washing my hands before I eat a meal, making sure that the utensils I use are clean, cleaning up, and having good food preparation habits. It's not really that difficult to do this, even when you're camping or traveling. When you're out camping, you can

find soap and water and carry it with you and use it. When you're traveling, you want to watch what bathroom you use, but you certainly can find public facilities that are clean.

About the only foods that I stay away from are things like crab meat, oysters, and clams.

Make sure your tap water is safe. Some communities have water systems that are contaminated periodically with a parasite called cryptosporidium. A call to your local water department should reveal whether this is a problem for you. If there's a chance that your tap water is contaminated, either use bottled water, bring tap water to a rolling boil for at least one minute, or install an in-home water filtration system.

You may have heard that it's not a good idea for transplant patients to have pets. Fortunately for everyone who loves animals—and that's most of us—there is no absolute prohibition against pet ownership, although there are definite precautions you must take. Transplant nurse Lisa Levin explains:

It's probably not a good idea to get licked in the face. And transplant patients should definitely never take care of any pet feces, whether they're cats, birds, or dogs. That's one of the benefits of transplant—you can legitimately say, "That's not my job." We give them permission to have pets with the understanding that any time you have anything in your house that's not you, you always have a risk that there can be disease transmission, or something carried on the animal that we can't anticipate. But we never ask people to give up their animals.

Long-term consequences of transplants

Your immune system doesn't only protect you from invaders from without, such as bacteria and viruses. It also protects you from subversion from within. Our own body's cells sometimes become abnormal, and multiply out of control. This is what happens in cancer. The normal immune system seeks out and destroys many cancers before they start. But when your immune system is suppressed, you're at somewhat greater risk of contracting all kinds of cancer.

Monitoring for cancer

Transplant patients should be especially watchful for signs of cancer. Women, for example, should conduct a breast self-exam once a month, and men should examine their testicles as frequently.

Both men and women should keep a close eye on their skin. Notice any suspicious changes in moles or birthmarks, which can be signs of skin cancer. It will be helpful to enlist your spouse in watching parts of your skin that you can't easily see—your back, for instance.

Your doctor should conduct tests to rule out cancer at least annually. Women should have mammographies and Pap tests, and men should have PSA (prostate specific antigen) tests. Both sexes should have fecal occult blood tests annually to look for signs of colon cancer.

In addition to detecting cancer, there are many things you can do to prevent cancer. Stop smoking. Eat a healthful diet and get plenty of exercise. Stay out of the sun, or make sure to protect yourself against sun exposure.

Jim Gleason describes what happened when he noticed several suspicious patches on his skin:

> Living with an immune-suppressed system does open one up to yet another danger: cancer. Those younger years of playing in the sun . . . would play a role in these later years now that the system was diminished. Yes, you are warned to stay out of the direct summer sunshine, but it really is too late. This summer I found several dry patches on my face that were diagnosed as pre-cancerous. With a simple freezing technique, these have been "burned off." It sounds a lot worse than it is—no pain, done right there in the doctor's office, a short process. A scab forms and drops off in a week or so. Hopefully they will not return. In my case, they still keep coming back so we repeat the process—no big deal. On the right forearm, it was another matter. This growth was biopsied and found to be the common form of skin cancer, and this had to be surgically removed. Surprisingly simple again. Local doctor's office, no pain (thanks to the local anesthetic), cut deep enough to remove it all, twelve stitches, and, "Sure, you can play tennis in a day or so"—a surprise. What little scar remains is quickly covered over by the hairy arm growth again.
>
> I do use the heavy SPF sunscreens any time I'm out in the sunshine for my walks or yard work. And of course there's the funny-looking hats,

but they do protect you from more of the same, right? Now I notice the many cautions from doctors and newsletters to have regular checkups with a dermatologist and wear hats and sunscreen—funny, I hadn't noticed them as much before.

Staying out of the sun is important not only to prevent skin cancer, but because some of the medications you may be taking, such as Lasix and certain antibiotics, can make you especially sensitive to the sun.

Post-transplant lymphoproliferative disorder

While all types of cancer are of concern to the immunosuppressed transplant patient, there is one type that is of special concern. It's called post-transplant lymphoproliferative disorder (PTLD), and as its name implies, it's a cancer of the lymphatic system that strikes transplant patients.

The cause of PTLD is not well understood, but it seems to have something to do with the Epstein-Barr virus (EBV) in combination with immunosuppression.[1] EBV is the cause of several different diseases, the most well known of which is infectious mononucleosis. In South African children, EBV has also been associated with a cancer called Burkitt's lymphoma.

PTLD strikes about 1 percent of kidney transplant patients, 2 percent of liver transplant patients, 8 percent of lung transplant patients, and somewhere between 5 percent and 20 percent of heart or heart-lung transplant patients. Children seem to be at particular risk of PTLD.

The disorder can arise within a year after transplant or not for several years. Since the lymphatic system is spread throughout the body, PTLD can manifest in many different ways, in the transplanted organ or outside of it, and the symptoms of PTLD are many and varied. The initial symptoms can range from a mild fever to sore throat to inflammation of the lymph nodes.

The main treatment for PTLD is an immediate decrease in immunosuppressive medication, which, of course, increases the chances of rejection. This is sometimes combined with cancer chemotherapy, antiviral medications, or other treatments. Although a large percentage of patients respond to treatment, this response, alas, is frequently temporary. While the majority of kidney and liver recipients with PTLD respond well to the withdrawal of immunosuppression, most heart recipients with PTLD will eventually succumb to the disorder.

Because of the poor prognosis associated with standard treatments for PTLD, you may wish to consider experimental treatments if you develop this disorder. As this book is being written, the National Cancer Institute is sponsoring several clinical trials of proposed therapies for various lymphoproliferative disorders, including a number aimed specifically at PTLD. You can find more information about these clinical trials by calling the NCI's Cancer Information Service at (800) 4-CANCER or by searching the PDQ (Physician's Data Query) database at NCI's CancerTrials site on the Internet: *http://cancertrials.nci.nih.gov/.*

This is not the place for a full discussion of cancer clinical trials. For a detailed overview, including information on finding, evaluating, and deciding whether to participate in cancer clinical trials, see *Cancer Clinical Trials: Experimental Treatments and How They Can Help You,* by Robert Finn (O'Reilly & Associates, 1999).

Living life

Did you get your transplant merely because you wanted to stave off death, or did you get it because you wanted to live a full life? We hope it's the latter, and we hope you'll take the comments of the following four people—a doctor, a nurse, and two transplant recipients—to heart.

Dr. Sharon Hunt says that some transplant patients have a hard time returning to a normal life:

> We make every effort to get transplant patients back to living a normal life. I give them the same advice I'd give anyone: clean living, exercise, eat right, don't get fat, control your blood pressure. To me, one of the biggest challenges is taking people who have usually been chronically ill for some years, and trying to convince them that they are normal, that they can exercise, become employed, go to school, and lead normal lives. That's a tough mind set to change for a lot of people. Some transplant patients travel the world, but most are pretty conservative about trying out their wings.

Nurse Lisa Levin points out that transplant recipients are welcome to travel the world:

> We've had recipients travel all over the place. We've had people in the Middle East, we've had people in Europe, we've had people go on

cruises. I think that when they pass the early post-transplant phase, and they're well, and they can support all their medications, and they have access to medical care, then I've never heard of anyone with any restrictions. The only thing that does come up occasionally is that travel to some places requires vaccine shots up front that may have live viruses in them, and that's not very safe. We do try not to have people do that. But otherwise there's no restriction on travel.

We spend a lot of time saying, "Listen, you did this because you wanted to improve your quality of life, and if these are things that you want to achieve, then we'll support you in any way that's safe."

Kidney-pancreas recipient Lori Noyes tells how much better she felt after her transplant, and how she has returned to a full working life:

I was on 60 or 70 pills a day when I got home from the transplant, but that was okay, because in the two or three years prior to the transplant I was already taking a lot of pills. I was a lifelong diabetic who was used to time schedules and medication. So for me it wasn't that hard. I know for a lot of transplant patients that kind of drug regimen is overwhelming. But I knew this is what I had to do to feel better.

I started exercising, and within four months I got rid of the cane, I started driving again, and I regained almost all the use of my legs. I'm still numb in my feet, but those were numb anyway for years. I was feeling better than I had since high school. I was free of insulin and non-diabetic. I didn't have those high-blood-sugar, low-blood-sugar mood swings anymore. I felt almost euphoric. I couldn't believe the difference, and I said, "Why didn't I do this years ago?"

Other than the side effects of drugs—extra hair growth, high blood pressure, and high cholesterol, all caused by the cyclosporine—I have been great, but I will never be as healthy as I was that first year. The main reason, I'm sure, is that I'm working. I'm under more stress. I do more things. I'm more like a normal human being instead of my euphoric honeymoon year. That was wonderful, but it's time to get back to real life.

Steve Rahn didn't let a little thing like a liver transplant interfere with his life:

It seems to me that the primary goal of transplantation, beyond the obvious life-saving objective, is the restoration of normalcy. Although individual circumstances vary, many recipients find themselves in much *better shape post-transplant than they ever were before. In my case, after five years of increasing disability and debilitation resulting from sclerosing cholangitis, a liver transplant at literally the eleventh hour not only saved my life but brought me to a level of health I had not known before. I was ready to go back to work full time within a couple of months of being discharged, but it took a while longer to find a job. Within six months of being transplanted, I was an active assistant scoutmaster in a Boy Scout troop that had at least one campout every month, all of which I happily participated in, and I stayed the whole week at summer camp with the troop. Less than a year after being discharged following the transplant, I went rock climbing and rappelling with the scouts. The following summer I had the honor of being elected as an adult to the Order of the Arrow.*

The standing joke when friends and I gather is for one of them to ask someone who doesn't know us to pick out the transplant recipient in the group. They invariably think it's someone else. As I said, this is not everybody's outcome. Your mileage may vary.

The Transplant Games

Perhaps the most triumphant expression of the transplant recipient's return to normality is the existence of the US and World Transplant Games.

The US Transplant Games are organized by the National Kidney Foundation and sponsored by Novartis Pharmaceuticals. Held every other year during even-numbered years, the event is a four-day athletic competition open to any recipient of a solid-organ or bone-marrow transplant. The 1998 Games were held August 5 to August 8 in Columbus, Ohio, on the campus of Ohio State University. It was apparently the largest gathering of transplant recipients in one place ever. The 2000 Games are scheduled for June 21 to June 24, 2000, at the Disney Wide World of Sports in Lake Buena Vista, Florida.

The World Transplant Games are held every two years during odd-numbered years under the auspices of the World Transplant Games Federation. The XII World Games were held September 4 to September 13, 1999, in Budapest, Hungary.

Recently, US and World Winter Transplant Games have been established.

For full information on both US and World Transplant Games, including application forms and travel information, contact the National Kidney Foundation at (800) 622-9010 or online at *http://www.kidney.org/recips/athletics/*.

CHAPTER 10

Emotional Responses

EVERY TRANSPLANT RECIPIENT—and every family member of every transplant recipient—experiences some degree of emotional turmoil. There's no way that a human being can go through such an intense series of events and remain untouched. It may be reassuring to realize that you're not abnormal if you have strong emotional responses in any stage of this process. You can lessen the stress on yourself and your family by knowing what emotional responses you can expect, and by learning strategies to help deal with those strong feelings.

This chapter looks at the range of emotional responses that transplant recipients and their families experience. First we'll describe the dizzying rush of emotions you have to deal with, and we'll pass on advice from professionals who have a great deal of experience in helping transplant patients cope. Then we'll take a look at the emotions you might experience while waiting for an organ, at the time of transplant, and during recovery. The chapter ends with a look at emotional impacts that may occur long after recovery from the surgery, including thoughts about your donor and your new organ.

The transplant roller coaster

It's difficult to imagine a series of events more emotionally trying over a longer period of time than the ones surrounding transplant. First there's the gradual—or not-so-gradual—decline in health and the depression that chronic illness often brings. Then there's the diagnosis of serious heart, lung, liver, or kidney disease, and those frightening words, "I think you may need a transplant." Then there's the long wait for an organ, the attendant anxiety about whether the organ will arrive in time, and perhaps guilt over the thought that someone must die so that you might live. When a living donor is a possibility, there's anxiety about whether someone will volunteer, and whether the volunteer will pass all her tests.

Then your pager goes off, and you rush to the hospital, all the while worrying about whether you or the organ may fail the last-minute tests. Then you wait in pre-op for the surgery to begin, a wait that often stretches for hours, plenty of time for your mind to conjure up all sorts of frightening or depressing scenarios. When you wake after surgery, there's often pain and discomfort, not to mention the side effects of high-dose immunosuppression. There's also euphoria, since many transplants leave the recipients feeling much better very quickly. But that euphoria can quickly be dashed by a serious complication, an infection, or a rejection episode.

Once the immediate crisis is over, and you're home from the hospital, there's the day-to-day tedium of caring for yourself and your new organ. Although your doctors will start reducing the doses of your immunosuppressive medications, troublesome side effects will likely remain. Although your transplant likely has left you feeling much better, you may have fears about working, traveling, or living life to the fullest, since rejection and infection can be ever-present worries. The term "emotional roller coaster" may be a cliché, but it's also an all-too-accurate description of the many feelings—and the rapid transitions among those feelings—that are part of every transplant experience.

Many transplant professionals believe that far too few patients and their families pay attention to the emotional turmoil that's a significant part of practically every transplant experience. As University of Chicago psychiatrist Larry S. Goldman, MD, puts it:

> One of the problems we see is that families and patients may minimize—or not even be aware—of how distressed they are, so they don't ask for the help. Or they may be ashamed or feel it may be too stigmatizing, so they don't request it.

It's important for you to put aside these feelings of shame. Be honest with yourself about the stress and the difficult feelings you might be experiencing. This is not the time to be stoic or to tough it out. You won't be taken off the list if you confess your fears to the social worker. No one will look at you funny if you ask to speak to the psychiatrist.

Unfortunately. it's not only patients and their families who ignore emotional problems. Dr. Goldman believes that members of the transplant team can easily fail to notice them as well. Sometimes, in fact, they seem to actually avert their eyes from potential problems:

If patients and their families come into the clinic and they're looking okay, and they're putting on a brave front, then the treatment team may not recognize the fact that there's a potential problem. The team may routinely say, "We've got psychological help available," but they won't necessarily urge somebody to take advantage of it. I think that there is a little bit of a dance on both sides to look the other way, and not see too much in the way of problems. And unfortunately, an awful lot of the situations that I've gotten involved in are things that hit a crisis because they weren't prevented or dealt with early. It would be much better if there were more resources and more willingness to use them on both sides.

In the following sections, we'll explore many of the emotional issues surrounding transplants, largely in the words of transplant patients, their families, and transplant professionals. See if you recognize yourself in these words.

Emotions during the wait

When you're told you may need a transplant, there's a flurry of activity. You meet with the transplant team, and you're evaluated medically and emotionally. Every part of your body—including your wallet—is poked and prodded. Finally you're told that yes, you're a transplant candidate, and yes, you'll be placed on the list. Someone hands you a pager, and you clip it to your belt, and you go home.

And you wait.

And you wait some more.

A month goes by, or two. Maybe a year goes by, or two.

The phone never rings. The pager never beeps. You change the batteries and phone the number yourself to make sure it's still working. Yup, it is.

It's the first thing your friends and relatives ask when you see them. "Any word?" "How much longer?" "Where are you on the list?" You have no answers, and when you ask those same questions during your clinic visits, the transplant team has no definitive answers either.

Meanwhile, your symptoms are worsening and your illness is progressing. You're worrying that an organ may not come in time. It's the mother of all stressful situations.

Mary E. Burge, a social worker on the heart transplant team at Stanford University and the Lucille Packard Children's Hospital, explains:

> The waiting period is so stressful because it's a time in which the much desired thing is out of a person's grasp. You have no control over when it's going to happen. Usually people learn from their parents or their teachers that if there's something you really, really want, you should make that your goal, and you should hitch your wagon to a star and go for it. But waiting for a donor is something you have utterly no control over. People who are used to having total control over their own lives, or who have had professions in which they're completely in control, such as airline pilots, usually have a very hard time coping with being dependent on circumstances, on some random act happening to somebody else. It's very difficult for some people to be dependent on others. Many men have a really hard time not being able to drive, if that's something they can no longer do. It forces them to be dependent on their wives for their connection to the outside world.

Ms. Burge describes coping techniques that people can find helpful during this waiting time:

> People need to keep their lives as balanced as possible to help them cope. I think people who just cancel everything and sit by the phone, or get obsessed with the beeper have a difficult time. People who are able to continue working in even the smallest way, so they can preserve that part of their identity, people who keep in touch with their friends, people who take walks on level ground, people who have pets to take care of or children to take care of usually have an easier time, because they can keep that sense of self esteem that comes from doing things for other people.

> Sometimes people who are more passive actually cope better with the waiting because they don't have the same habit of feeling as though they're in control. They can just go with it. Religious faith is helpful to a lot of people. For people who are believers, attending church or synagogue can be very useful. Sometimes meditation can be very helpful or learning relaxation techniques or learning self-hypnosis.

> It's also good to just talk about what's on your mind. Talking about difficult, anxiety-provoking subjects just makes it feel not nearly so bad. That's one of the reasons the support groups are so successful at helping

people cope. People reinforce each other's coping. Having somebody you can call if you start losing it is very helpful. The people who attend the support groups are actually more compliant afterwards, because the groups tend to foster doing well—taking your medicine, eating properly, getting exercise. I think people really need to band together and help each other out.

Cardiologist Randall Vagelos believes that it's important for anyone awaiting a transplant to get out and live life, and not worry about waiting:

In general, unless they're in the hospital deathly ill, my recommendation has always been not to sit around and wait for the transplant. For these patients, life is too precious to be wasted. They may never get offered an organ, or they may have a poor response to transplantation. Fifteen percent of [heart] patients who are transplanted, at least across the board in the world today, will be dead at the end of the first year. So one has to make sure that these people know that they have to take every day and enjoy it or make the most of it.

Attitude

A positive attitude is heart recipient Jim Gleason's defining characteristic. Even as he was waiting in the hospital for a new heart, too ill to be sent home, Jim wrote:

What comes next, we will have to wait and see. Everybody asks: "How do you feel about all this, Jim?" Very positive, as it turns out. It does seem like quite an exciting adventure in front of us all. As the patient, I feel I have it the best, with those around me going through the really tough worrying part. . . . Recent weeks of being very tired and weak make one appreciate the "old self" much more. The promise of a new Jim really does seem too good to be true. When my dad died of congestive heart failure at the same age back in 1970 (he was born with a congenital heart problem), these options didn't exist. We really do live in an age of miracles.

As mentioned previously, you can read *A Gift from the Heart*, Jim's detailed account of his heart transplant, at *http://transweb.org/people/recips/experien/gleason/*.

You can choose—it really is a choice—whether to regard this experience as an exciting adventure or as a terrible calamity. The events may unfold more or less the same way no matter what your attitude is. Optimism isn't going to make your time on the waiting list any shorter, and pessimism isn't going to make it any longer. But a positive attitude will probably make the wait a good deal more pleasant, and pessimism will probably turn it into a miserable ordeal.

Guilt

During the wait, many transplant recipients find themselves experiencing uncomfortable thoughts about the source of their organ. Some people feel intense guilt about the fact that someone must die so that they may live. In the words of kidney-pancreas recipient Melanie Horne:

> I know that for myself at least a couple times the thought passed through my mind, "Why me? Why do I deserve this? Somebody has to die. If someone else doesn't die, I will." These thoughts do get you sooner or later. Somewhere in the experience it will hit you. The reality is, it's a lottery. Either you get it, or someone else does. Somebody's going to die somewhere in the long run.

Chapter 14, *Donors and Recipients*, discusses the complex interplay of emotions in the donor/recipient relationship.

Depression

It's hard to maintain a positive attitude when you have end-stage liver or kidney disease, congestive heart failure, or a serious lung condition, and you're waiting for a transplant. A certain amount of depression is quite normal in this situation.

Many potential transplant patients have a psychological condition that's technically called reactive or situational depression. This condition is considered an "adjustment disorder." An adjustment disorder is a counterproductive reaction to a stress—such as serious illness—that's characterized by an impairment of function greater than one would normally expect. Unlike major depression (also called clinical depression), which we'll discuss in a moment, reactive depression typically gets better once the stress is relieved.

But this doesn't mean that reactive depression should be ignored. Psychiatrists are trained to distinguish between an ordinary case of the blues, reactive depression, and major depression, and they're highly skilled at prescribing medication, when necessary, to relieve the symptoms. Sometimes medication isn't necessary, and a few conversations with the psychiatrist or other psychotherapist will be all that's needed. If you or a family member are feeling depressed, you should definitely seek an appointment with the psychiatrist attached to the transplant team.

Rae Ann Berry, a social worker in Stanford University's liver transplant unit, points out that most of the patients admitted to her unit may have a diagnosable adjustment disorder:

> Most of our patients, but not all, are evaluated by a psychiatrist, and some of our patients are on antidepressants. We like them to go through our psychiatrists here, and we want to be sure that the psychiatric medications they are prescribed are the ones that are the kindest to a sick liver. There are certain kinds of things that people are going to have depression about, if it's getting through to them at all. You could probably say most of our patients have an adjustment disorder. And it doesn't all have to be plastered over with drugs. But we really do carefully assess that, and when we see the need, we have those medications.

Psychiatrist Kathy L. Coffman, who works with transplant patients at St. Vincent Medical Center in Los Angeles, says that patients with reactive depression often don't require medication:

> It depends how severe their symptoms are. If they're depressed because of their disease or because they're worried about the transplant, a lot of times just sitting down and talking about transplants helps them incredibly. And that's true whatever the organ is. I had a gal referred to me a couple weeks ago and talked with her about transplant. She had been somewhat depressed, and we talked about changes in her medication because she was already on antidepressants. When I called her back the following week to see how she was doing, she said that she couldn't pinpoint what it was that we had talked about that made her feel better, but she felt much better and she wasn't sure she really needed to increase her antidepressants.

A major or clinical depression is another kettle of fish. Major depression is a serious psychological disorder that's characterized by a severely depressed mood and loss of interest in all the normally pleasurable things of life, such as sex, food, friends, and entertainment. In addition, someone with major depression will have at least three of the following symptoms:

- Poor appetite or significant weight loss or weight gain

- Inability to sleep (insomnia) or sleeping excessively (hypersomnia)

- A marked agitation or retardation of movement

- Feelings of hopelessness

- Fatigue or loss of energy

- Feelings of worthlessness or excessive guilt

- Diminished ability to think or concentrate

- Recurrent thoughts of death, fantasies of suicide, or actual suicide attempts

While you were reading through that list you probably noticed that some of those symptoms are identical to the symptoms of liver, kidney, or heart disease. Others, when not carried to extremes, are normal consequences of living with serious illness. That's why it's difficult to self-diagnose major depression. A psychiatrist experienced with transplant patients must be the one to make the determination. Dr. Goldman says that one thing he's learned in his career as a psychiatrist is that making this diagnosis can be critical:

> Picking up on a clinical depression is very important because, first of all, their whole medical risk goes up for almost any condition, let alone transplant. The prognosis is much worse if they have a major depression. And the other thing is that there will be reasonable concerns about whether the person will have the energy and motivation to recuperate from the surgery.

Fortunately, even major depression can normally be treated with great success by antidepressant medication and psychotherapy, and a diagnosis of major depression will not by itself disqualify a patient from consideration for transplant. Dr. Coffman says that she's aware of no good scientific studies proving that major depression alone causes higher mortality in transplant patients. This is important for both doctors and patients to recognize, since patients sometimes try to mask their psychological symptoms for fear that a diagnosis of depression will affect their standing on the list. On the contrary, being open about these symptoms is more likely to result in effective treatment that in turn will lead to a better transplant experience.

Emotions at the time of transplant

The pager beeps, you rush to the hospital, you're put through the last-minute tests, and then you expect to be wheeled directly into the operating room. But often transplant patients wait for hours before that happens. As we've seen in previous chapters, there may be several reasons for that wait. Before the organs are retrieved from the donor, several different transplant teams have to arrive at the donor site, and they have to coordinate their surgeries. If you're waiting for a kidney, you'll likely have to wait for the heart and liver teams to finish first. Then the team has to travel back to your hospital, and they have to prepare the organ for transplant.

Meanwhile, you're being prepped for surgery, with anxious friends and family hovering close by. As kidney-pancreas recipient Lori Noyes recalls, this period can be awfully trying:

> It's funny, the wait on the list was no big deal to me. I didn't get jumpy with the pager or anything like that. But the long wait the day of the surgery was probably the toughest. Everybody around me was so excited and trying to call, and I said, "Everybody, just chill out! Because if you get all freaked out, I'm going to start freaking out." I tried to remain calm by telling everybody not to talk to me, except for my parents. I was scared, though.

If you find yourself experiencing a lot of anxiety while waiting for the surgery to begin, don't hesitate to bring this to your nurse's attention. Often it will be possible for you to take a tranquilizer to help you calm down. You may also ask to speak with the social worker or the psychiatrist. Sometimes the anxiety can be the result of a lack of information. Occasionally the transplant team may simply forget to keep you informed about the reason for the delay. If that's the case, just keep asking for updates.

Once the transplant operation starts, you will be anesthetized, and you won't have to worry about a thing until you wake up hours later. Not so for your friends and family members anxiously waiting for the operation to be finished. The minutes can seem like hours, and every hour that passes can seem like an eternity.

Usually, surgical teams are very sensitive to the needs of the waiting family, and either they'll phone out with progress reports, or they'll send one of the team members out every so often with news. Family members may want to inquire about this before the operation begins. You may want to ask:

- How long will the operation take?
- How often will you provide updates?
- Who will be providing those updates?
- Will we be able to wait in a room of our own, or will we be sharing a waiting room with other families?
- Should we make sure to stay in that room, or can we take a break for a meal?
- If it's going to be an especially long operation, would you suggest that we go home for several hours?

John Best remembers his wife Suzan's liver transplant very vividly:

> I'm a weird person. Things really don't bother me all that much. But when she was in surgery, I finally had a chance to break down, and I broke down hard. I broke down when she went in. Her parents had left to go to a motel room and I stayed up for forty-two hours straight. I couldn't sleep and I just became a walking zombie. There was another transplant there at the same time as hers and that one only lasted six-and-a-half hours. Suzan's lasted sixteen hours. I was desperately worried.
>
> But there was one doctor, an intern, who kept me informed of the progress, which made me feel a little bit better about it. But I was still worried that he was lying to me. She lost quite a bit of blood. Her doctor finally came out and told me that she was still in surgery and that he lost count after he gave her her thirtieth unit of blood. He said that he was knee deep in blood.
>
> That made it even worse and I was still trying to hold all my emotions back, and it was getting more difficult. Then when I saw her finally, she came wheeling out, and she just looked dead, and it choked me up, but I was holding it back because I wanted to go in there and see her. When I finally went in to see her, that's when I broke down again.

Recovery in the hospital

The period immediately after transplant can be a very confusing one for the patient. The residual effects of anesthesia can interfere with memory, for example. Often people will have no memory of detailed conversations they've had with family members, doctors, and nurses in the first 24 hours or so after surgery. This can be pretty disconcerting for everyone involved. Family members shouldn't worry about this, since it's normal and to be expected.

The patient may well be experiencing discomfort from the surgery itself and from some of its consequences. For example, if you're on a ventilator, there will be a tube down your throat. Not only can it be very unpleasant to have a machine breathing for you, but you'll be unable to speak. But that doesn't mean you can't communicate. You'll usually be given a pencil and paper, and though you'll be weak, you'll probably be able to communicate in writing. If there's no pencil and paper handy, make writing motions with your fingers. Someone will get the message.

Adding to the confusion will be the side effects of high-dose immunosuppression, notes Dr. Goldman:

> A problem that we see in the early post-op period is that fairly commonly people will get confusion or delirium from some of the medications. Prednisone is notorious for that. It can cause big mood swings, and it can make people very, very goofy. But some of the other immunosuppressants can do it too. Actually, just being that sick, being in the intensive care unit for a while, losing blood, and all those sorts of things can cause problems [with mental orientation].

> How we treat this depends on what kind of goofiness they're having, and whether they have any awareness of the problem. I've seen people who have had very peculiar psychotic experiences such as hallucinations, but they know it's not real. They almost immediately realize it's from their medication and they don't act on it. I saw a patient once, for example, who thought there was a fire outside his sixth-story window, and this was going on for days, but he was still a very calm guy. He didn't tell anybody about it, he didn't say anything, and he didn't react to it. So it wasn't a problem, and we didn't need to do anything. On the other hand, if the patient doesn't know where it's coming from, is getting very anxious or worked-up, is starting to pull intravenous lines out, or is starting to talk to the voices he's hearing, then we have to intervene by changing the medicines they're on. Sometimes we give them some tranquilizers to calm them down, and sometimes we do some other environmental manipulations.

Dr. Coffman finds that some transplant patients ascribe their emotions to the organ itself, and not to the drugs they're taking:

> Initially, people may be euphoric from the steroids because they're on a high dose. As they taper it down about the end of the first week, a lot of patients get quite weepy and more emotional, and some of the men will say, "I know you gave me a woman's heart." If they say that to me, I'll go back and check. That's a pretty rare happenstance, because most women's hearts are not big enough for a big male. And I'll tell them, "No, your donor was male. Remember I told you before the transplant that when you cut the steroids back you can get that weepy feeling?" It's like when women have their babies and their hormone levels drop, they get a little weepy for a few days sometimes. I try to educate them about that.

Dr. Coffman emphasizes that she checks on the sex of the donor not because she believes that a female heart can indeed make a man more emotional. On the contrary, she does it to reassure the recipient that his emotions are more likely due to his medications.

Patients and their families need to realize that even when the surgery has gone well, and the recovery seems to be proceeding apace, the emotional roller coaster ride likely still has a few surprises, a few stomach-turning twists and turns, left in store. Social worker Rae Ann Berry explains:

> Right after transplant when a patient wakes up, and we're telling him that it went well, there's such relief on everybody's faces and they smile all the time. There's just huge relief, and we know that that euphoria is only going to last a day or two, because there's going to be some kind of little blip. Things don't just get better, better, better, and it's over. There's the day when they're running a fever, there's the day when they may be in rejection, there's the day when we're not sure a blood vessel is hooked up right, or whatever. You haven't seen depression until you've seen somebody who waltzes out of here with a big smile on his face and maybe that night something happens and they have to come right back to the emergency room.

Dr. Goldman points out that transplant recipients often get overly upset in the face of medical setbacks. An understanding psychiatrist can be of great help in that situation:

> A lot of the post-transplant emotional issues are directly proportional to how well somebody does medically or surgically. People who sail

through the surgery, who have no complications, who seem to be tolerat-
ing their medications okay, who get out of the hospital fast, those folks in
general don't have a lot of psychological problems. People who are in the
hospital for a long time, who have a lot of complications, those folks can
get awfully beaten down. The more problems you have, or the longer the
problems go on, the more likely you are to see some kind of emotional/
psychological reaction to it that's going to be problematic.

I do not routinely get involved with everybody post-operatively. The
ones that sail through have no need for me. I'm more likely to get called in
for the ones who seem to be having a lot of problems. Mostly I see people
getting depressed and demoralized. They start losing some of their opti-
mism. And sometimes people who have difficult personalities will start
squabbling and having more difficulty getting along with the nursing staff
and other members of the medical team.

The biggest problems are mostly people sort of curling up and giving
up. These are the ones that are really problematic, but fortunately it
doesn't happen very often. We try to find some way to re-instill some hope
while being realistic. Sometimes they have just misinterpreted several set-
backs as being more ominous than they really are. Sometimes we can be
of help pharmacologically. There are some medications that may help pick
up their mood, at least transiently, and get them back on track again.
Sometimes it's a matter of just rallying some extra support, bringing in
more family members or a minister or whomever.

Long-term emotional responses

Transplants also have emotional consequences that can extend well beyond
the immediate recovery period. Some transplant patients seem almost afraid
to live their lives, an issue discussed in Chapter 9, *Living with a Transplant*.
Dave Souza, who rapidly resumed an active life in the months following his
kidney transplant, nevertheless expresses anxiety about his medical future.

I know part of the fear is the future, not that my future is clear. I
mean, physically there are doubts, because they tell you that each year
you have the kidney your chances of rejection grow greater, statistically. In
the past, it used to be mostly elderly people who needed kidney trans-
plants. So the statistics weren't that good in your favor of keeping it for a

long time, because they would die of natural causes within five to fifteen
years of their transplant. Nowadays the figures are getting different.

> *The doctors' attitude is, "Hey, if you lose that one, we'll get you*
> *another one," and it's a little bit cavalier, but that's the way they see it,*
> *that's their job. For me, I would be crushed if I lost my kidney. I was in a*
> *dilemma when I had that mild rejection. I was really scared that all of this*
> *good work by everybody was going to go down the tubes, and I'd be back*
> *to square one. It was a frightening specter.*

> *And I think the future at any point during the process is what scares*
> *most people from making the right or wrong decision. I feel, still today,*
> *that I made the right decision in going for the transplant, but it didn't*
> *make most of the pluses or minuses go away—they're still there. I may*
> *get cancer. I may get a bad infection.*

It's worth mentioning that it's not just transplant recipients who fear cancer or a bad infection. Those illnesses, and many others, can strike anyone at any time. Not one of us is guaranteed good health indefinitely. In fact, none of us is guaranteed a single moment beyond the moment we're in. You can choose to worry about your health constantly, or you can choose to live fully while recognizing that life is filled with uncertainty.

Some transplant recipients find themselves obsessing about their organ and its donor. Occasionally this takes a lighthearted—and perfectly healthy—form. Sometimes people name their organs, for example. There's a fellow who regularly participates in the TRNSPLNT email group (which will be discussed in Chapter 11, *Family and Support*) who describes himself as "home of Sidney the Kidney."

In many cases, however, joking and lightheartedness can mask a very deep discomfort about having someone else's organ residing within one's body. Dr. Coffman says that such issues arise more commonly than one might think:

> *We are, after all, kind of primitive beings, as much as we try to think*
> *we're sophisticated. Some patients are concerned that they may take on*
> *the personality of the donor, but I've never found that to be true. When-*
> *ever people think they've taken on some qualities of the donor I try to go*
> *back and find out what the ideas are, because people have a lot of funny*
> *ideas.*

Sometimes people get the idea that if their spouse has a heart transplant they won't love them the same with somebody else's heart. We've had patients who were concerned because they thought if they got a heart from somebody who wasn't saved, it might jeopardize their own salvation. I've had patients who thought if they had a kidney transplant from their son who was gay, it would make them gay.

Probably a great many transplant patients do have these ideas and don't voice them. If they do voice it, it comes out in humorous ways. They think if they get a heart or liver that's from a different ethnic group they'll start eating a different kind of food, or they say that they hope they get the heart of a young stud so they'll be more manly. It's probably a lot more prevalent than people are willing to admit, and most of the time it comes out as humorous.

Although some of the thoughts that might arise about your organ may seem embarrassing, you should discuss them openly with members of the transplant team. Taken to extremes, these obsessive thoughts can have negative physical consequences. As an example, Dr. Coffman recalls two patients who got the erroneous idea that their organs came from Native Americans:

I deal with it straight up. If they have questions about it, I'll tell them what my experience has been over twelve years. We had a patient once who for whatever reason had a strange idea that his donor was Native American. He thought he had had a vision of the donor's family standing outside the room. He got the idea that if he had a Native American heart that he shouldn't take white-man medicine, and he should only take herbs. We actually had another patient who got that same idea for whatever reason, and actually stopped his cyclosporine and got a bad rejection—and this was an educated person. For the patient who had the vision, I went back to see who the donor really was and whether there was any evidence that this donor was Native American, and found out that the donor was not Native American. He was a blond surfer-boy kind of guy. The organ was not even retrieved at the hospital where the transplant took place, so the whole fantasy that the donor family was outside the window looking at him was totally in the recipient's mind.

Finally, it's important for all transplant patients to remember that while a new organ may well change your life for the better in many ways, it won't restore you to the state of perfect health you may have enjoyed before you were struck by serious illness. The failure to recognize this fact can be responsible for a great deal of disappointment, self-destructive behavior, and emotional turmoil. Conversely, those willing to face this fact head-on are most likely to have a satisfying, long-term post-transplant experience, says Joan Miller, a transplant coordinator in the Department of Cardiothoracic Surgery at Stanford University Medical Center:

> Heart transplant recipients make a big transition from being heart failure patients, and many patients believe that when they get their heart they're going to be well, and they're going to be able to put illness behind them. But really what they've done is they've changed their diagnosis. They're not heart failure patients anymore, but now they're immunosuppressed. And they may feel better, and may have a longer lease on life, and be able to go back to work and do things that they couldn't do before, but they're still tethered to the medical system. They still have to have lab tests done and come see the doctor. And that's a hard transition to make. I don't know that they really deal with that beforehand, because then they were really focusing on day-to-day survival.

> It's a hard adjustment to face when they get out of hospital. They take a lot of medicines that have multiple side effects. Some are good, some are bad, some are really absolutely rotten. And it's very stressful. They're often living with a family member in an apartment a block from the hospital for a couple of months in the sort of intense relationship they haven't had with anybody in years. Spouses start to bicker. Relationships between moms and children start to fall apart. I think they all need somebody they can talk to who can listen to them and help them deal with this, and help them come to grips with the fact that, yes, it's hard, and yet there are some good things that come from it—and there is life after transplant.

CHAPTER 11

Family and Support

THE TRANSPLANT ROLLER COASTER is the name sometimes given to the emotional turmoil that surrounds organ transplants. The transplant recipient is not the only one on that roller coaster, of course. The recipient's entire family is along for the ride, especially the primary caregiver, who is often a parent or spouse. Children also feel these emotions acutely, and they may have more difficulty in dealing with them than do adults.

In this chapter, we'll discuss how the transplant experience affects couples, children, and whole families, and we'll point you to some of the many avenues for emotional support. The section on couples will also be useful to anyone who serves as the primary caregiver for a transplant patient, whether or not that person is your spouse.

A number of resources for support will be mentioned throughout this chapter. Full contact information is listed in the appendix, *Resources*, at the back of the book.

The couple

Serious illness changes the entire dynamics of a relationship. While almost every married couple vows to stay together "in sickness and in health," the constant strain of an extended illness can wear down even the strongest of ties. On the other hand, struggling through this adversity can also bring a couple closer.

Michael Browning and his wife Julie looked into this issue when deciding whether to list their infant son Morgan for a heart transplant.

> What I've heard is, if your marriage is doing well, this will make it stronger, and if your marriage is struggling, it'll make it weaker. And we had a pretty good relationship. This was our first son, and we'd been married about two years, and things at my work were really going well, Julie's

business was going well, and most other things in our lives were in pretty good shape at the time.

As noted in Chapter 2, *The System*, family support is one of the most critical items assessed by social workers in initial evaluations. Kidney-pancreas recipient Melanie Horne cautions:

> *Don't do it alone. You've got to have your family with you. If you don't have family, you've got to have your friends with you. If you don't have friends, you'd better get some. I did it alone the first time. My family is back in New York, and they didn't care anyway, and I hadn't been here long enough to form a whole lot of bonds. I'm a fairly strong person, and the nurses had told me that I am the only person that they've seen come through the transplant unit who went through it without support and came out alive.*
>
> *A lot of places won't even list somebody without support. But because I'm fairly tough, they did list me. Initially, though, their reaction was not to list me. They put me before this panel of psychologists who said, "How are you going to deal with this without your mother or father?" "Well, the same way that I've dealt with the rest of my life without my mother and father." I just brushed it off, and they realized that I was kind of tough. But this time around things have really changed. I've got my husband Chris now. I know this is going to be a whole lot different than the first time around. A lot easier. I sure wouldn't want to have to do it without him.*

If you don't have someone who can serve as a primary caregiver, who can nurse you 24 hours a day and seven days a week while you're waiting for a transplant and through recovery, you may not even get listed. And it's not just physical support that the patient needs.

Liver recipient Suzan Best explains:

> *You have to be able to talk to somebody. You have to choose the right person to talk to openly about it, somebody who will listen to your heart, somebody who will support you no matter what. If it weren't for my husband I really doubt I'd be here talking to you. You need somebody there for you all the time, especially when you get sick. Some people, it seems to me, they hear you, but they don't listen to you. Perhaps there was a time in my life when I was reaching out, and nobody reached out for me, to*

> help me mentally, emotionally, or physically. It's important to have some-
> body to lean on, and to trust that they will be there no matter what. I
> went into denial, and I also got depressed, but right before the transplant I
> was kind of accepting the fact that I could perhaps not make it. You go
> through a lot. But when you have somebody supporting you that you can
> talk to openly, it helps a lot.

Caregiving around the clock is an enormous responsibility for a single
human being to assume. If you don't have regular respite, it can become an
overwhelming burden. Think about the ordeal John Best endured during his
wife's two-year bout with liver disease. A roofer, John suffered an accident
just before Suzan became ill. This was fortunate, in a manner of speaking,
because he spent those two years unable to work and receiving disability
insurance payments. This allowed him to spend all of his time taking care of
his wife:

> My advice for other caregivers is to hang tough. When patients are
> very sick before the operation, they build up a lot of anger because they
> don't know why this is happening to them, and there are many days when
> the patient can't do what they need to do. There's sadness, depression, and
> you have to make them eat whether or not they want to. Basically you
> just have to have a lot of patience.

> And you have to know their medications. That's especially important
> because that's going to keep them alive until the transplant. Make sure
> you keep all the medical appointments, and most important, I found, is to
> keep track of the paperwork. I took down her vitals. I wrote down when
> she ate, and when she urinated and how much. I wrote down when she
> had a bowel movement, and what it looked like, and how much. I just
> kept a current record so every time we saw the doctor we could show
> whether she was getting better or worse or was stabilizing. When she was
> bedridden for awhile, I would turn her over and bathe her quite thor-
> oughly. It's very important just to be clean, because that makes them feel
> just a little better about themselves.

If you're going to be the caregiver, the thought of providing this level of care
may seem overwhelming or even impossible. But nurses or other members
of the transplant team will teach you what you need to know to care for your
loved one. And if you really can't do all that, your insurance may pay for
some home nursing care.

If you find yourself in the caregiver role, you may be able to keep your sanity by keeping your eye on the light at the end of the tunnel. Eventually an organ will become available, the transplant will happen, and after a recovery period the recipient will become much more self-sufficient.

Suzan finally received her liver transplant three weeks before she and John were interviewed for this book. John had a sound of great relief in his voice when he said:

> I've been taking care of Suzan 24 hours a day for roughly two years. Now that Suzan has had her transplant, I'm probably going to take one more month off work. Maybe only two more weeks, because she's quite capable now of taking care of herself.

But then he went on to say:

> It's going to be hard for me to separate now from being a caregiver.

The dynamics of a relationship can be altered, depending on who is ill and who is the caregiver. Mary Burge, a social worker at Stanford University's heart transplant unit explains:

> There's often a kind of relationship role reversal. It can get especially stressful in the "classic" marriage where the husband is the main person dealing with the outside world and the workplace, and the wife is at home. If the husband is no longer able to work, and the wife maybe needs to go out and get a job, that's very stressful. [The couple] really needs to listen to each other and talk to each other and not take things for granted. I encourage people to talk about what they think is going on, and not expect the other person to read their mind, but to say what's on their mind.
>
> And they shouldn't be afraid to ask for what they need emotionally. Both caregivers and patients sometimes need to say, "I need a hug," or "I need a back rub," or "I need an evening off," or "I need to spend some time with the boys (or the girls)."

Time off is an especially precious safety valve for caregivers. The pressure of being on duty all day, every day can easily wear a person down in no time. If you're in that position, you owe it to yourself—and to the person you're caring for—to take occasional breaks. Perhaps a relative can take care of your spouse or child one or two evenings or a week. Perhaps your insurance plan will provide an occasional visit from a home healthcare aide. Perhaps you qualify for "respite care" through a local social service agency. The person most likely to know about such things is the social worker on your transplant team.

Psychiatrist Kathy L. Coffman points out that the stresses surrounding transplant can doom a relationship if the couple is not careful:

> We've seen couples that stayed together during the whole illness and transplant, and after the recipient healed the spouse said, "Okay, I stuck with you through that, but this is it, I'm out of here." Sometimes couples will pull together, but once the danger is over, they're out of there. We see that particularly with patients that may have had marital problems before, or when there was alcohol abuse or drug abuse in the family. They really had washed their hands of the person, but decided to stick around to help out just to make sure the person survived.

On the other hand, Dave and Linda Souza are living examples of the observation that good relationships can get better when tempered by the fire of illness and transplant. They think that Dave's long bout with kidney disease and his subsequent transplant have on balance made their 25-year marriage stronger, although they acknowledge that there have been strains:

> Dave: The strains have been my reactions to the pills more than anything else. But I think the experience has both kept us in touch with how much time we really have together, and that the quality time should be there all the time. I know I appreciate her and the support I got through the whole thing, as a friend as well as a wife. And it made me more aware of my own shortcomings, because they're under a microscope even in my own mind. I mean the pills don't make me oblivious to how I react. They make me very keen on how I react, and then I get mad at myself, which kind of escalates the reaction.

> Linda: I think early on, the way he accepted dialysis and how he took care of himself added to my love and respect for him, because it was something that, to be quite honest, I didn't think he could handle. And this is something he had to do four times a day, and he was still able to keep working, and I've been in awe of that. And then it also brings your friends and your family together. We experienced so much love and support from family and friends.

Dave: Yes, a lot of people—even some friends that I thought were very lukewarm towards me—actually came up to the hospital unexpectedly.

Linda: I was overwhelmed by the love and friendship of family and friends, too. And then the experience just makes you appreciate life more and realize how precious it is. And I think it's made us stronger human beings. You don't realize quite how big a deal it is until other people bring it to your attention and say, "Oh, my God, you went through a transplant?"

Dave: Our walks together are better. In the past, we'd take walks together, and my wife is very energetic and likes to walk fast. Especially when I was on dialysis, I was a slowpoke. So it was like, "Hey, you up there, you want to walk with me?" But the walks that we would take after the transplant I thought were much more meaningful, and we both could compromise on the pace.

The following is a list of suggestions for couples that can help keep a relationship strong throughout the transplant experience:

- Expect this experience to alter your family dynamics.
- Be open with your partner about your feelings.
- Don't expect your partner to be a mind reader. Tell him or her what you need.
- Pay close attention to your partner's feelings.
- Keep your eyes on the prize: a successful transplant and recovery.
- Whether you're the patient or the caregiver, expect to feel anger, impatience, resentment, and other unpleasant emotions occasionally. This doesn't make you a bad person.
- In the face of such emotions from your partner, be understanding. Recognize that these emotions may be side effects of the medications or the disease process or the strains of being a caregiver.
- If you are the primary caregiver, take frequent breaks. Find an alternate caregiver so you can take evenings or entire days off occasionally.
- Find things about your partner to admire as he or she copes with this adversity.

- Recognize that once the patient has recovered, family members may experience a flood of uncomfortable emotions that had previously been held in check. This is normal.

- Whether you are a transplant patient or a family member, do not be afraid to seek outside support.

Children

This section discusses how children react to transplants in parents or other family members. Chapter 12, *Transplants in Children*, focuses on family issues when children are patients.

Psychiatrist Larry S. Goldman thinks that transplant families should pay especially close attention to their children:

> When families find that they're starting to have more quarrels, more tensions as a unit, or any individual is starting to get more depressed or anxious out of proportion to the circumstances, that should be a pretty clear warning that something is going on. And you've got to pay attention to everybody in the family. We tend to think of just the adults in the family as the ones who are affected, but sometimes the kids are the canary in the mine. They're the early-warning system that something's wrong. A kid who's not doing well at school or who's acting out suggests that there may be some systemic problem that needs to be looked into.

Paying attention to the children should start from the beginning of any transplant experience. As Dr. Coffman explains:

> Children are often left out of the discussions, and they have a lot to say about how the transplant's affecting them. I always encourage people that if their children have questions, they should bring them in to the clinic. Give them an opportunity to ask questions as well. We have coloring books for the kids [that help explain transplants], and I often talk with the kids.
>
> We also try to make sure they let their teachers know that one of the parents is being listed for a transplant, so they can make it into a project for the class. It could be some kind of a book report or some kind of talk about transplant stuff. Depending on the age of the child, it can generate

a lot of discussion at school, and that way the children can get some sup-
port from their classmates, who will know what they're going through.

When there are several children in the family, one of whom needs a transplant, the healthy child is sometimes pushed to the side. This is what happened in JoLayna Arndt's family. JoLayna donated part of her own liver to infant son Ashton, and this had some unfortunate consequences for Jordyn, her three-year-old daughter:

> *It was awful for my daughter Jordyn. More than anyone, she suffered the most emotionally. She was away from us for three weeks. (She stayed with her aunt, who is wonderful.) When you have a child that is sick, the thought of losing him is just overwhelming, and I wanted to make sure that I didn't regret one minute of Ashton's life, so I spent a lot of time holding him before the transplant.*

> *As I look back, I was obsessed with Ashton, and it was very difficult to tune into Jordyn's needs and how scared she was. I did the best I could—I didn't neglect her. But emotionally I was with my little boy. It took me four months after the transplant to realize this, so it was probably eight months of me not being a really in-tune mom. She was having a lot of accidents. She was wetting a lot, and she was really emotional and very insecure, and she's not an insecure child. She's a very outgoing, dramatic child. So I met with a child psychologist by myself, and I talked to her about it, and I've just made changes since then.*

> *Jordyn's done really well, but there are still some effects that are lasting. She is more insecure than she was before, and I think in a way she had to grow up a little too fast during that time.*

> *She knew what was going on. We told her that Ashton was very sick, and she had to know that he could be gone. She came to the hospital to visit him, and see how awful he looked when he was in ICU. I questioned whether we should bring her to the hospital and see him like that. The psychiatrist persuaded me by saying that children are very intuitive. It's better if she's involved. So I did let her see him in ICU. When she came to visit me at the hospital after I donated part of my liver she wouldn't get near me because I had lots of equipment all around me.*

> *It's very hard on Jordyn. Ashton receives a lot of attention still because of his transplant. For months after the transplant, when people*

would come to the door they wanted to see him, not her. And that's really hard on her self-esteem.

When someone in the family is very ill, children can become so concerned with how upset their parents are that they may suppress their own feelings. Although deep down they're probably extremely worried and unsettled, they may not want to express this for fear of upsetting their parents more than they already are. For this reason, you may get the impression that your children are coping reasonably well, when in actuality they are not. To avoid this problem, the adults in the family should share their own fears and feelings with the children and encourage the children to reveal theirs as well.

Children are creatures of habit and routine, and a serious illness can turn family routines upside down. When someone is sick, children may focus more on interruptions in these day-to-day routines than on the health of the person who's sick. They may fuss about, "Who's going to choose my clothes in the morning?" "Who's going to drive me to baseball practice?" "Will Daddy make dinner every night now that Mommy's sick?" While these concerns may seem trivial or insensitive to you in the face of a life-threatening illness, children need to be assured that the world is not falling completely apart, and you should soothe them with the thought that while their routines may need to change somewhat, they will be respected as much as possible.

If you give your children room to feel their own fears about the sick person, and if you respect their need not to worry about their routines, you will be going a long way toward helping them cope with this family crisis.

The following is a list of suggestions for parents to help them provide the extra emotional support children might need when a family member is facing a transplant:[1]

- Healthy children can often be pushed aside and ignored during a family crisis like this. Pay special attention to these children.

- Watch for warning signs in your children, such as regressive behavior (e.g., toileting accidents) or problems in school.

- Keep close tabs on all your children, even the ones who seem to be coping very well. Excellent coping may mask some deep-seated fears.

- Help your children maintain their routines.

- Encourage your children to ask questions about the illness.

- Encourage your children to express their fears and worries about the illness.

- Inform your children's teachers about what's happening, and suggest that they discuss transplants with the class.

- Be a model of the type of behavior you desire. If you talk respectfully and take time-outs when angry, your child will learn to do likewise. If you scream and hit, that is how your child will handle his anger.

- Seek professional help for behaviors that trouble you.

- Teach your child to talk about her feelings.

- Listen to your child with understanding and empathy.

- Be honest and admit your mistakes.

- Help your child examine why she is behaving as she is.

- Distinguish between having feelings (always okay) and acting on feelings in destructive or hurtful ways (not okay).

- Have clear rules and consequences for violations.

- Discuss acceptable outlets for anger.

- Give frequent reassurances of your love.

- Provide lots of hugs and physical affection.

- Compliment your child for good behavior.

- Recognize that disturbing behaviors can result from stress, pain, and drugs.

- Remember that with lots of structure, love, and time, problems will become more manageable.

The family

We like to think of ourselves as autonomous individuals, but everything we do affects everyone around us. When serious illness and the possibility of a transplant enter your life, one thing you can count on is that your entire family unit will change in ways that are extremely complex and difficult to predict. As Dr. Goldman explains:

> Most transplant teams will work very closely with the family right
> from the beginning, because they realize that this is an issue that affects
> the whole family system. There's sort of a ripple effect: whatever the

psychological reactions are in the patient, everybody in the family has to deal with it. There may be financial implications, time implications, child-care implications. So the transplant team typically will have a social worker get involved to get a good handle on what the family is like—how they deal with stress, what kind of strengths and weaknesses they've got—and try to anticipate any rough spots and work with them ahead of time. One of the advantages of having a waiting time before a transplant is that you have a chance to intervene and help people prepare so that things don't go awry later on.

When one member of a family is ill, it's easy for the healthy ones to ignore their own needs in their understandable desire to care for their loved one. But such intense focus on one individual can backfire. Families need to broaden their focus, to recognize that even in the midst of a crisis everyone in the family has individual needs that must be met. As transplant coordinator Joan Miller puts it:

Sometimes it's easier for the patient than it is for the family. I think the families need somebody they can go to and say, "He's driving me crazy! I'm going to kill him if he does so and so one more time!" They're supposed to be sweet and supportive and understanding, but nobody's listening to the family because everyone's focused on the patient.

Dr. Coffman points out that family problems sometimes appear after the main crisis is over:

When they're waiting for transplant, a lot of times the family is in crisis mode, and they do what needs to be done at the time. Oftentimes what we see is that after the transplant, once the patient is doing pretty well and getting ready to be discharged, then the spouses and the family members come in and say, "I don't know what's wrong with me. I was fine during this whole thing, but now I'm crying. I think I'm losing it. Is this normal?"

We sit and talk about that because often once the recipient is safe, the spouse or other family members can let down that front they've been keeping up of being strong for the patient. It's their turn to go through the process emotionally of allowing themselves to express all the fear, and the worry they had that they were going to lose the person. Also, sometimes they have a lot of anger that they formerly weren't able to express, because it's not always acceptable to voice that anger and resentment for the burden you bear of taking care of someone.

Getting support

If this book has a single message, it's that no one can go through a transplant alone, and that every transplant patient needs support. Support from your family is wonderful and absolutely necessary, but one of the silver linings behind the cloud of serious illness is the myriad opportunities out there for emotional and social support from a much wider community. When you're a transplant patient, it's as if you've been admitted to membership in an exclusive—but rapidly growing—club whose members are only too happy to share their experience and their knowledge.

Support can come in many forms, from formal appointments with psychiatrists and psychologists, to support groups organized by your transplant team or outside groups, to Internet-based discussion groups, to religious organizations and extended families. Explore the various support options, and participate in the ones that seem to fit the best with your needs and your personality.

In the early days of transplant surgery, practically every patient was given a thorough evaluation by a psychologist or a psychiatrist who was permanently assigned to the transplant team. While this does still happen in some transplant programs, it's becoming increasingly rare. As transplant coordinator Joan Miller explains:

> I think patients need more emotional and psychological support than we give them. But we get into funding issues. We've tried over the years to have psychologists or psychiatrists as part of the team. But the reimbursement is inadequate, and so they don't stay because they're not getting paid, and nobody has the money to pay them. I think that patients need more help adjusting to everything that's going on than is possible for us to give them. But it's a dead-end street. I've been here a long time, and I've seen people try many different things and none of them have worked. Also people are very resistant, and even when they really need it, and we refer them to see somebody, they often don't want to go because of residual stigma.

Dr. Coffman thinks that it's easy for medical professionals who deal with transplants every day to forget how traumatic the experience can be for patients:

> It's true that in some programs the patients do not get much teaching or support as to what to expect with transplants, particularly with certain

organ types. I think with kidney transplant patients you see that often, because it is considered such a routine surgery nowadays. A lot of kidney transplant programs don't think it's necessary to have a psychiatrist involved unless the patient may have had a history of psychiatric problems or a history of drug abuse or alcoholism.

I think that's a mistake. There's a big transition going from being healthy first of all to depending on a machine with all the issues of dependency and loss of control that implies. Then you have the prospect of waiting on a list if you don't have a living related or even a living unrelated donor, and that prospect can stretch out even for years, depending on the blood type and tissue type. Then you have to try to resume an active life after transplant. Generally people are expected to go back to work after they get their kidney transplant without having been taught about the different phases of that process or even knowing much about the side effects of the medications. I think that's a lot to expect someone to negotiate emotionally without some kind of support.

What I always tell my patients is that we've seen hundreds of transplants done, but for them it's sometimes their first experience with major surgery, and many of them are facing the prospect of death if the organ doesn't come in time. That's very stressful.

Rae Ann Berry, a social worker in Stanford University's liver transplant team, has long experience working with transplant patients, and she's a great believer in support groups. She urges all of her patients, both pre- and post-transplant, to come to the support group sessions she organizes twice a week, every week. She encourages them to bring any questions they have, and she also encourages them to bring along family members, especially the primary caregiver:

I think the one thing patients and their families can do to make the experience as pleasant as possible is to open themselves up to other people in the same situation. For some people that is so very hard. They want to keep their illness a secret. They don't even want to tell their family. But it's really harder to deal with when you're not talking about it. And it's much easier to talk about it with people who are going through the same thing. This is why we found that it really does a lot of good to require the patients to come to a support group when they're here for the evaluation.

That connects them with a community they didn't even know existed. That connection makes a huge difference. Sometimes people get on the phone and talk for hours about their symptoms, comparing what they've been through.

For eleven years now I've led a support group every Monday and Thursday, which are the same days the patients come for clinic. For some of our patients, part of the contract is that they will come to the support group once a month or whatever, because some people are in denial about the seriousness of their illness. They think, "I'm not really that sick. I'm going to change my diet and get well." They aren't really facing what they're dealing with, and so they really get a dose of reality in these groups.

There are a million different ways to do support groups, and they all work, but the way that works best for me is to have the pre- and post-transplant patients and their families in the same group. Before a transplant, patients and their families are scared to death. They don't know what to expect, and they don't know what a transplant patient looks like afterwards. And for them to be in a room with people who have been transplanted, it's like, "Maybe this is not the calamity I thought it was."

Ms. Berry recommends that parents bring their children to support groups:

I encourage people to bring their children, even rather small children, because sometimes those kids they hear the words "liver transplant," and they also hear that Daddy or Mommy is sick, but you can't always look at a liver patient, especially until they get really sick, and tell that anything's wrong with them. Kids don't always exactly believe it. And then when the patient gets really sick and the kid is thinking about it, sometimes what they fantasize about what is going to happen is so much worse than reality could ever be, that it just helps. I like younger kids to come to these meetings once at least. Older kids sometimes come once a month or so.

Patients have a lot to contribute to each other, says Ms. Berry:

I'm really careful to not turn a support group into a class, because I want the patients to learn as much as they can from each other about what it feels like to go through this, and what this experience is like. I always tell them that nobody who works on this service, not the doctors, not the nurses, not the social workers, has had a liver transplant. We don't know what it feels like. We don't know what the drugs feel like. So they have to learn those things from each other. I always call the post-op patients the experts. Someone will ask a question and I'll say, "You've asked a question that needs to be directed to an expert. Suzan, can you answer that?" So they learn from each other. I especially don't let medical people visit because it would definitely turn into a question-and-answer session with the doctor or nurse.

Suzan and John Best attended some of Ms. Berry's support-group meetings, although not until after the transplant. As Suzan explains:

Before the transplant I wasn't going to any support groups. I couldn't go anywhere. I was too sick. I would have needed a wheelchair, and I couldn't sit for more than half-an-hour. I would have had to lie down. But since the transplant my husband and I have gone to support groups. We've only been to a couple, but I believe that they did help. It helped me knowing that I'm not the only one. It doesn't matter what age you are or anything, there's understanding, and hope, and family, and friends, and people who are going through the same thing. It kind of gives you hope.

Not every support group is organized the way Ms. Berry organizes hers. Joan Miller explains that in Stanford's heart and lung transplant programs the support groups meet only once a month. Many of those meetings are topic-oriented, with a member of the medical staff presenting information about specific subjects, such as organ procurement or the side effects of immuno-suppressants.

If you don't care for your transplant center's support group, or you just want to attend another independent group, check out the Transplant Recipients International Organization (TRIO). Among TRIO's many wonderful services is a network of support groups open to all transplant patients and their families.

TRIO is structured as an association of individual member chapters, of which there are at least 50, with many more in development. It is these individual chapters that organize local support group meetings.

You can find additional information on TRIO or TRIO chapters by contacting the national organization at (800) 874-6386 or online at *http://www.trio-web.org/*.

The excellent TransWeb site maintains a long list of support groups that includes the TRIO group among many others. You'll find that list by searching at: *http://www.transweb.org/*.

The Chronimed mail-order pharmacy (*http://www.chronimed.com/*) prints an annual directory of support groups. For a free copy, call a patient specialist at (800) 888-5753.

Dr. Coffman points out that you can't always predict what will happen at a support group. If you attend only one meeting, you may hit a day where the rest of the group is feeling pessimistic, and you may come away feeling worse than when you arrived. On another day, that kind of group may fit your mood perfectly, and you'll come away feeling relieved that you are not alone, that other people are as worried as you:

> You get different kinds of people coming to transplant support groups, and depending on who shows up on a given night, the group may have a very different tone. Some of the patients will say, "People are only allowed to talk about the positive things in support groups," whereas if they come on another night they may say, "Oh, people are only talking about the negative parts of transplants." So you can't please everybody with support groups.
>
> And some people are just not joiners, whether that's going to church or other kinds of social groups. Some people are just not comfortable in group settings. Sometimes people are more comfortable if they are going to get information, rather than if there's no set topic. And for other people it's the other way around: other people like to sit and talk about what's going on, and want tips on coping with chronic illness and support for the caregiver. I think it's a very individual thing.

Dave Souza would probably agree. He seems to have the same attitude about joining support groups that Groucho Marx had about joining clubs. Groucho, you'll recall, joked that he wouldn't join any club that would have him as a member. Dave explains that he didn't need psychological support, and he preferred not to get the kind of social support he'd find in a formal support group:

> I did go to the psychiatrist at [one hospital] and the psychologist at [another], and they both said, "You seem pretty well balanced. Give me a call if you need us, and as far as I'm concerned, we don't need to schedule you for any more appointments." The other groups, the group therapy and so on, I just always thought of them as a social thing, and I didn't want my situation to be a social thing. I see too many times where people

*get together and their only common ground is the transplant. And I
wanted to be social with people but not because of a physical malady.*

Dr. Coffman agrees that formal support groups don't fit every patient's personality. She points out that there are some perfectly acceptable informal alternatives:

> *Often we try to hook people up into a buddy system. If they are interested but don't want to come to a support group, we'll try to introduce them in clinic to people who are about their same age and have had a transplant. They have a chance to ask questions about what it's really like, patient to patient.*

Melanie Horne has had some truly remarkable success with her informal hospital contacts with other transplant patients:

> *More than anything else, the most valuable tool is the other transplant patients you meet in hospital. You meet while waiting for your labs to be drawn. In fact, I know a girl who got a KP [kidney-pancreas transplant] a couple months after I did, and she met a guy who got a heart transplant, and they're married now. I met my husband [when I was] at the hospital for my second transplant anniversary. They gave me a whole slew of things to do, and one of them was to get an EKG, and he works in the cardiac diagnostic department. We were married at the home of another recipient who was transplanted a couple months before me. His wife was my maid of honor, and yet another kidney-pancreas recipient was our minister. It was a KP party!*

Some transplant patients are fortunate to have a wide network of friends, or they may be members of highly supportive religious communities. Such networks are invaluable aids when you are ill. Don't be reluctant to make use of them.

Heart recipient Jim Gleason has a particularly supportive group of friends:

> *What happened after I was told I'd need a heart transplant was a whirlwind of phone calls to family and friends. Networks of researchers responded with articles and facts that were very encouraging. The prayer chains were unbelievable—from many different faiths and congregations. Wills were written, priests seen for anointing of the sick, finances put in order, work materials turned over to a super supporting . . . team of friends, insurance companies contacted, etc.*

JoLayna Arndt's religious community provided both physical and spiritual sustenance:

> Probably the best source of support was our religion. We're Mormons. Our ward was wonderful to us throughout the whole thing. Before the transplant we had a fast—you go without food for 24 hours—and they dedicated a fast for Ashton and myself. The whole neighborhood fasted for 24 hours, and they prayed during that time. Our religion was probably the best source of support for us, and not only spiritually. They brought us meals for three months following the transplant. They shoveled our sidewalks, because there's lots of snow here. We were well taken care of, and that's probably why we didn't need to seek psychological support.

Support on the Internet

Support needn't come only in face-to-face meetings. The Internet is an excellent source of support for organ transplant patients. There are email lists and Usenet newsgroups and real-time chat forums that provide a wealth of information and support. Dr. Coffman cautions that as good as these groups are, you will find both accurate and inaccurate information online:

> Patients who are not comfortable going to any kind of group often look on the Internet. I always tell them to be sure and ask us if they have questions about things they find on the Internet because some of things I've found there have not been particularly accurate. That's of concern to us, especially if there's anything on the Internet that has to do with people's medications or discontinuation of medication. People have to be cautious to not accept everything they read or hear from the Internet or other sources.

By far the best source of support for organ transplant patients and their families on the Internet is a mailing list called TRNSPLNT. The easiest way to subscribe to this mailing list is to point your web browser to this address: *http://www.concentric.net/~Holloway/*.

An alternate method is to send email to: *listserv@wuvmd.wustl.edu*. In the body of the message type the following single line (substituting your name): SUB TRNSPLNT Jane Doe.

Once you subscribe to the list, your email box will fill with impassioned and informative messages on every aspect of organ transplants, contributed by people who are in the trenches: patients, their families, and healthcare providers. You'll find discussions on dealing with the side effects of medications, advice on traveling to foreign countries, first-person accounts of transplant surgeries and rejection episodes, information about new scientific developments, and informed discussions of the politics of transplantation. You'll even find creative ideas on what to do with all that extra hair growth induced by cyclosporine. Once you join TRNSPLNT, posting questions or comments of your own is as easy as sending an email message.

The TRNSPLNT email list is generally very productive and congenial. While tempers do flare occasionally, especially when the discussion turns to issues of organ procurement and distribution (see Chapter 2 for more on these controversies), in general participants in TRNSPLNT are considerate, pleasant, and well informed. The TRNSPLNT list proved to be the single most productive source of information and ideas in researching this book. A number of the people quoted in these pages make regular, eloquent posts to this list.

Messages sent to the TRNSPLNT list are "echoed" in the Usenet newsgroup *bit.listserv.transplant*, and vice versa, messages sent to that newsgroup appear in the email list. Some people find it more convenient to access the discussions through Usenet. Usenet is a collection of more than 20,000 "newsgroups" on every conceivable subject. While providing full instructions for participating in Usenet newsgroups is beyond the scope of this book, you can do so by using "news reader" software that's included in software from America Online and in full-featured Internet browsers such as Netscape Communicator and Microsoft Internet Explorer. You can also access Usenet newsgroups through a web site called Deja.com: *http://www.deja.com/*.

A huge archive of past TRNSPLNT discussions is available by sending email to *listserv@wuvmd.wustl.edu* with the following single line in the body of the message: INDEX TRNSPLNT.

In response, you'll receive an email message containing instructions on requesting monthly compilations of all TRNSPLNT discussions going back to 1994.

One of the most valuable aspects of the TRNSPLNT list is the massive Frequently Asked Questions (FAQ) document, compiled by Mike Holloway, the list moderator. You'll find many of your questions about transplants answered in this document, currently available in four parts. In fact, much of the rest of this chapter is based on information found in the FAQ. The FAQ is posted to

TRNSPLNT and to *bit.listserv.transplant* every few weeks, and it's also available at: *http://www.faqs.org/faqs/medicine/transplant-faq/part1/*.

While TRNSPLNT is clearly the dominant online support group for those interested in organ transplants, there are several others as well.

A list called txlongterm is intended for people who have been transplant recipients for extended periods. It concentrates on rehabilitation and unique physical issues for such people. To subscribe to txlongerm, go to: *http://www.onelist.com*.

The DIALYSIS list is specifically for kidney patients. To subscribe, send mail to: *listproc@mail.wustl.edu*. In the body of the message type the following single line (substituting your name): subscribe DIALYSIS Jane Doe.

If you are a spouse, family member, or caregiver of someone who is awaiting or is already a recipient of a lung transplant, you may wish to subscribe to the ASSIST mailing list. To do so, send email to: *ASSIST-request@HOME.EASE.LSOFT.COM*. This message will be read by a real person, not an automated list processor. In your message, include your loved one's diagnosis, describe your relationship to that person (e.g., spouse, parent, sibling), and mention whether the person has already been transplanted or is waiting.

The Second Wind National Lung Transplant Patient's Association maintains a discussion list for messages concerning lung diseases, lung transplants, problems, solutions, and "life in general." You'll find the subscription form at: *http://www.2ndwind.org/join.htm*.

If you are dealing with the long-term complications of years of diabetes, even after a kidney/pancreas transplant, you may wish to subscribe to the Kidney/Pancreas Support Group. To subscribe, send a blank email to: *kptx-subscribe@makelist.com*.

Some mailing lists are so busy, and some topics generate so much discussion, that it's not unusual for an email discussion list to generate more than one hundred messages each day. To avoid having all these messages overflow your mail box, subscribe to the digest version of the list if it is available. A digest subscription will give you a single message that contains the full text of all the previous day's individual messages. Instructions on switching to the digest vary from list to list. Normally you'll find these instructions in the welcome message you receive when first subscribing.

In addition to *bit.listserv.transplant*, there are several other support groups on Usenet that may be of interest to people in various transplant communities:

- *alt.support.diabetes*
- *alt.support.diabetes.kids*
- *alt.support.heart-defects*
- *alt.support.hepatitis-c*
- *alt.support.kidney-failure*
- *sci.med.cardiology*
- *sci.med.diseases.hepatitis*

If you prefer more immediate interaction in online support groups, consider participating in one of the many real-time chats available through various online services. America Online has the most extensive list of scheduled chats, but other services—including some that do not require special subscriptions—host transplant chats as well.

For an up-to-date list of scheduled weekly chats organized by service, see the TRNSPLNT FAQ, described above. A listing of chats for a sample week at the time this book was written includes the following groups:

- America Online
    - Sunday, 10:00 p.m., Kidney/Pancreas Transplant
    - Monday, 8:00 p.m., Donor Awareness
    - Monday, 9:00 p.m., Liver Disease & Transplant
    - Tuesday, 9:00 p.m., Lung Transplant
    - Tuesday, 9:00 p.m., Bone Marrow Transplant
    - Tuesday, 9:30 p.m., Kidney/Pancreas Transplant
    - Thursday, 7:00 p.m., Heart Transplant
    - Thursday, 9:00 p.m., Bone Marrow Transplant
    - Friday, 8:00 p.m., Kidney Disease & Transplant
    - Friday, 9:00 p.m., All Organs/Tissues Transplant
    - Saturday, 9:00 p.m., Parents of Bone Marrow Transplant Recipients
    - Saturday, 12:00 midnight, Organ Transplant Support

- Prodigy
  - Thursday, 9:00 p.m., Transplants
  - Friday, 9:00 p.m., Transplants
  - Saturdays, 9:00 p.m., Transplants
- Microsoft Network
  - Wednesday, 10:00 p.m., Transplant & Diabetes

The Children's Liver Alliance currently hosts four separate chats rooms for adult family members, children (including siblings), medical professionals, and staff and volunteers. For more information, email: *Livers4Kids@earthlink. net* or call (718) 987-6200. To find out more or to participate, go to the Alliance web site at: *http://www.livertx.org*.

If you have access to ICQ—special software that allows for real-time chats over the Internet—you may wish to register your ICQ number at the Organ Transplant Support Group Chat, *http://www.jensoft-cs.com/icqlist.html*. Visiting this web page will allow you to contact about 100 transplant recipients (at last count) who have indicated a willingness to chat about their experiences.

There are several things that are important to remember about any patient support group, whether it's an email discussion list, a Usenet newsgroup, or a real-time chat. One is that you should take everything that's said in these groups with a large grain of salt. While many participants are well-meaning and well-informed, some are misinformed, others have axes to grind, and a few are actively malevolent. Double-check everything.

Occasionally long arguments, called "flame wars," break out in these groups. Some of these flame wars descend into insults and personal attacks. On other occasions people with, shall we say, idiosyncratic ideas shout loudly to be heard. Some participants are snake-oil salesmen, whose shameful *modus operandi* is to peddle their quack remedies to vulnerable and desperate people. Thankfully, these unpleasant individuals are a relative rarity on most transplant-related groups.

Nevertheless, you should enter these support groups equipped with healthy skepticism and a good suit of flameproof armor, or you may find that they do more harm than good. Used properly, they can provide not only valuable information, but also a community of like-minded individuals who are going through what you're going through.

JoLayna Arndt even managed to get a free consultation from a transplant surgeon she found on the Internet:

> The Internet was a wonderful source. You're able to ask a lot of questions to parents of children who had already received liver transplants that you're not able to ask your doctors or you don't think to ask your doctors. I did a lot of research about liver transplants on the Internet. I was able to communicate with one of the best surgeons in the country involved in pediatric liver living donations. I was able to email him, and make sure he thought the surgeon we were using was okay. He looked at Ashton's liver numbers and made sure he agreed it was the time for a transplant.

Dr. Goldman points out that it's important to place information you gather from other transplant patients, on the Internet, or from other sources, in the proper context:

> In general, I'm a pretty strong believer that the more information you get and the more sharing you do, the better off you're going to be. The downside, of course, is that sometimes you hear horror stories that aren't buffered or put in the right perspective, or you get misinformation.

CHAPTER 12

Transplants in Children

CHILDREN ARE NOT MINIATURE ADULTS, so there are some special considerations regarding transplants in children. This chapter will examine some of these unique factors. We'll begin with some suggestions for dealing with a sick child. Next we'll tell the story of two new parents as they waited for a heart transplant for their infant. We'll discuss important options for children who are candidates for liver, kidney, and lung transplants. We'll conclude with suggestions for helping a child live with his transplant.

Please note that this chapter does not endeavor to be a complete guide to dealing with a seriously ill child who requires hospitalization. For that we recommend the book *Your Child in the Hospital: A Practical Guide for Parents (Second Edition)* by Nancy Keene and Rachel Prentice. It is small, but over-flowing with excellent suggestions and information.

Another good source comes from the Stadtlanders Pharmacy web site (*http://www.stadtlander.com/transplant/childtx.html*), where there's an informative collection of articles on children and transplants.

Two other sites concentrate on children with liver disease, but contain material of interest related to all pediatric transplants. You'll find the Children's Liver Association for Support Services at *http://www.classkids.org/*, and the Children's Liver Alliance at *http://www.livertx.org/*.

Dealing with a sick child

How a child and her parents deal with transplant depends to a great extent on the child's age. Infants and toddlers won't benefit too much from pre-transplant teaching, for example, but they will benefit from having family members keeping them company in the hospital as much as possible. Famil-iar toys and videotapes will also help the child feel at home, and if she has a special "blankie," keeping that item with her will increase her level of comfort. Although as a parent you'll be feeling a great deal of anxiety, it's important to remain positive and to keep from communicating that anxiety to your child. Even very young children are adept at picking up emotional cues from their parents.

As social worker Mary Burge observes:

> *Parents are really torn between wanting to extend their child's life and wanting to protect them from any avoidable pain. Parents really suffer when their children are getting poked.*

Preschoolers will definitely benefit from pre-transplant teaching, but since they have such a poor sense of time it's difficult to know when to begin this training, especially if they may be waiting for an organ for several weeks or months. You'll want to explain the procedure in play, by using dolls, and they may also benefit by seeing some of the actual instruments that will be used. After transplant, be sure to keep the incision covered with bandages, since children at this age tend to be very sensitive about the intactness of their bodies.

School-age children (six to twelve years old) can be given quite a bit of pre-transplant teaching. You'll be able to teach them something about their disease, and they will benefit from tours of the hospital room, the operating room, and the intensive care unit. They may also want to speak with doctors, nurses, and other people who staff these areas. Making things concrete in this way is important, because children at this age often imagine scenarios that are far worse than reality. On the other hand, school-age children may also deny the seriousness of their illness. It's important to be explicit and completely honest with them about exactly what will happen, where the tubes will be, how long the incision will be, what sort of discomfort they're likely to feel after the surgery, and so on. Although you may be tempted to downplay these matters, the child may lose his trust in you and in the medical team if you do.

Adolescents should be given as much information as you would give to an adult. As anyone who has ever read J. D. Salinger's *The Catcher in the Rye* knows, teenagers are exquisitely sensitive to the slightest hint of dishonesty or phoniness.

Teenagers are in the midst of making the difficult transition into adulthood, and as Ms. Burge explains, serious illness can interfere with that process:

The role reversal can be very difficult for teenagers, because they're just getting independent, and all of a sudden they're thrown back into more dependence on their parents than they would like.

Because of the importance of body image to teenagers, the side effects of immunosuppressive medication can seem particularly devastating. As discussed previously, these side effects include weight gain, acne, and excessive hair growth. Even the levels of such bodily changes that normally come with adolescence can be upsetting to a teenager, and the increased levels that come with immunosuppressive medications can tempt teens to gamble with cutting down on their drugs. It's critical to acknowledge this openly and to emphasize the consequences of organ rejection.

With children of all ages, it's important to make sure they understand what you've attempted to teach them. After you've taught them, make sure to ask them to repeat back what they think will happen. You may be surprised by some of their misconceptions. Encourage them to engage in discussions, and answer all their questions honestly and completely with age-appropriate explanations.

Encourage your children to confide in their friends about their transplant experience, and encourage those friends to write, to phone, and to visit your child in the hospital. This will provide welcome peer support.

The transplant experience

It's frightening to think that your child has an illness so severe that he might need an organ transplant. There's no way to prepare yourself for the emotional turmoil that can result. You'll find some suggestions for dealing with the powerful emotions that can arise in Chapter 10, *Emotional Responses*, and Chapter 11, *Family and Support*.

Michael Browning and his wife, Julie, experienced this fear soon after the birth of their first son, Morgan, in 1993. Julie experienced a normal pregnancy, but had a somewhat difficult delivery because of Morgan's relatively large size at birth. Since Morgan had some trouble breathing, he was sent to the neonatal intensive care unit (NICU) just after he was born.

The first indication that something was seriously wrong came when the neonatologist detected an odd-sounding heart rhythm. As a precaution she recommended that Morgan undergo an echocardiogram, which is an examination of the heart using sound waves. The test revealed that Morgan was suffering from hypoplastic left heart syndrome, a condition in which part of the infant's heart is seriously underdeveloped. Not too long ago, this condition was invariably fatal, so the new parents were devastated with the diagnosis.

Then someone mentioned that a transplant might be a possibility. Although Mike is himself a PhD neuroscientist with a broad knowledge of biology and medicine, he didn't know much about transplants, and the initial information he was given turned out to be inaccurate:

> The hospital where Morgan was born was not very knowledgeable about transplants. They told us we would have to go to Loma Linda Medical Center in California in order to get a transplant, and the idea to us seemed just appalling. It meant we would have to move our whole family from Denver to California while we waited. I didn't know much about the transplants at all, and what I did know was mostly in old people, and they just seemed very sick. We didn't know how successful it would be, and it sounded like a lot of surgeries for our kid. It just didn't seem to us like a viable option, and nobody at the hospital or our pediatrician seemed to think it was a good option either. So in the first hours after having heard the news we were basically planning to bring him home and have a few days with him until he succumbed.

> But then a cardiologist, whom we had never met before, showed up. He took us into another room and said, "Well, what have you heard?" So we told him what we had heard, and he told us that most of that was wrong. He started telling us, first of all, that the person who had originated pediatric heart transplants at Loma Linda was now chief of cardiology at Children's Hospital in Denver.

> The cardiologist told us that the major problem was keeping the children healthy enough until they got the heart. That was the first barrier we would have to get past. But for children who are reasonably healthy at the transplant, the surgery is quite straightforward, he told us. Almost all make it through the surgery fine, and then something like 90 percent make it to one year and five years. He said that when it's successful the children have virtually 100 percent heart capacity.

> We had been prepared for the down side of transplant, but were totally unprepared for the up side, which in our mind is relatively

unlimited, as far as Morgan's future is concerned. I went from thinking that my son was going to die in three days to feeling ecstatic 20 minutes later. I don't think we've looked back, ever, even though I must say there were very scary times waiting for the transplant because kids do get sick when they're not getting a full blood supply.

Waiting for an infant donor organ is just as difficult as waiting for an adult organ. Mike, Julie, and the medical team all worked as hard as they could to keep Morgan as healthy as possible for as long as possible, since there was no way to tell when an organ would become available:

We sort of got into a routine. The people at the hospital were really accommodating. They called him "Bubba" because generally in these neo-natal intensive care units there are just preemies, and he was huge—8 pounds, 15 ounces at birth. They also had sick kids in there and we needed to keep him as healthy as we could. He wasn't immunocompro-mised at that point, but he was weak, and if he had an infection of some sort when the heart became available, they might decline him. So we had to keep him healthy, as healthy as we could. We finally got our own little room within the NICU, which was great.

When Morgan was about three weeks old he became unable to breastfeed because he was just too weak. Then [Julie bought a breast pump and] we started on the bottle, and he was able to do that a little bit. We would measure the amount that he drank and then they would sup-plement it with breast milk given through a feeding tube. We were really trying to keep his weight up, since the bigger and healthier they are when they go for the transplant, the better. He actually gained almost a pound waiting for transplant.

We would be there for all the feedings except for the two overnight feedings. I was in a position where I basically didn't have to go into work. So Julie and I would just come in every three or four hours during the day and then take a break in between and go home. We could bathe him, and he was awake and could even smile. It's possible, as the father, that I had a closer relationship to him than I might otherwise have had if he had been normal and come home, and I had gone to work. But here I was, seeing him every three hours of every day for 41 days. That's how long we had to wait.

During that time, the doctors were giving Morgan medication intended to keep his heart as healthy as possible until the transplant. Unfortunately, the wait wasn't all smooth sailing:

> There were a number of crises that happened. Some little ones were based on just blood levels. This or that blood level would get a little bit out of kilter. So I would always look at the chart when I came in in the morning, to see if everything was okay. As soon as we woke up, we'd call the nurse and see what kind of night he had. It was really great to hear in the morning that he had a great night, and always tough when he had a tough night.
>
> The other, bigger challenge was the IVs, which were his lifeline. You know, he was a little guy, and the IVs just don't stay around long. They lose the veins, and then they have to get another one. During the course of this, they finally had to do what are called cut-downs. That's where they cut right in the inside of the elbow, to expose the deeper, bigger veins. It's stressful when they do that. And even that failed toward the end. They had to do another surgery where they go into the jugular vein in his throat, and thread an IV tube down closer to his heart. That required general anesthesia, and when he came out of that, he was on a respirator. That was scary to us because the kids who are on respirators have a harder time getting out of the hospital after the transplant, just because they're sicker. But fortunately he was able to be weaned off the respirator.

Finally, after 41 days, an organ became available, and the donor was very close by:

> As it turned out, there was a fairly good circumstance for us, because the donor child was on life support at Children's Hospital, and she had been declared brain-dead. Her mother had agreed to donate her organs, and I think two other children also got organs that same time from the same child. They were able to actually have her side by side with Morgan when they did the surgery, which was a good prospect, so we didn't have to worry about any problems in terms of time and the heart.
>
> They began the surgery around three or four o'clock in the afternoon, and we just sat in the waiting room for about five or six hours. The transplant coordinator—a great nurse whom we really love—came out about every 30 or 40 minutes to let us know how things were going. She

would tell us the next stage, so we could anticipate what was going to happen. I remember she told us one time, "The heart is in, and now they're going to try to warm him up and start the heart." Everything went fine. It was fairly uneventful, if you can call a transplant an uneventful surgery. There weren't any problems that they told us about.

Then about one o'clock in the morning we got to go in and see him. Of course he was on a respirator, but he had this rosy color for the first time since he was born, which was great. He moved fairly quickly to the transition intensive care, and we actually went home eight days later.

Morgan's continuing story is a happy one. As this is being written, he's a healthy and active six-year-old, with a completely normal younger brother and two very grateful parents.

Transplant options

If your child needs a heart transplant, your only option is to wait for a cadaveric donor. But if she needs a kidney, liver, or lung, a living donor may be a possibility. As transplant surgeon Michael Wachs, MD, of the University of Colorado Health Science Center, points out, the possibility of living donation in liver transplants has solved a major problem in pediatric transplants:

Because of the availability of living related liver transplants, the mortality on the pediatric waiting list has decreased dramatically. In other words, children really don't have to wait that long for liver transplants anymore, and fewer die while waiting. It has pretty much solved the waiting list problem for children.

Still, living donation is not the only option, says Dr. Wachs:

I present parents with three different options for pediatric transplant. They can get an organ from a child who dies—a whole-organ, sized-matched transplant. Or they can have a cut-down or split-liver transplant from an adult cadaver donor. Or they can go through living donations. I set all three as possibilities, and that way the family doesn't feel pressured if they, for whatever reason, can't go ahead with a living donation. They don't feel that they've abandoned their child, or that there are no other options.

> *The ultimate decision is left up to the medical doctors and surgical doctors based on the urgency of the patient's condition. The first one of these that we ever did in Denver was for fulminant [sudden and severe] hepatic failure in an eight-year-old boy. We waited for twenty-four hours trying to find a cadaver donor for him, and when one was not available and his condition was deteriorating, the father volunteered to be a living donor. In other situations, you could have a child who can wait a year or two in stable condition if they're not deteriorating medically, so you can tell the parents, "We can do an evaluation and think about you as a potential donor, but let's give the kid a little while on the waiting list, and see if we can get a cadaver donor first, so we don't have to put you through the donor surgery." It really depends on how the kid is doing and what the family situation is.*

Similar considerations apply to children needing kidney and lung transplants as well.

Living with a transplant

Anti-rejection medications have similar side effects in children as they do in adults. As previously mentioned, children can have particular problems with these side effects, especially as they enter their adolescent years.

Not every child experiences serious side effects. As Mike Browning explains, his son's worst problem is an overgrowth of his gums, which is a common side effect of cyclosporine:

> *Morgan has some excess hair on his arms, and some on the back of his neck, and his sideburns are longer. Instead of stopping at the top of his ear, they go down to the middle of his ear. But he has no hair on his face or his chest.*
>
> *He does have trouble with gingivitis, though. He really has puffy gums, and we're working with gargling and flossing and things like that. There's no decay or unhealthiness; it's just that it's less attractive. He may need to have periodontal surgery at some point, although the transplant team has a lot of luck with Listerine gargles causing the gums to retract. His gums are healthy, but they're just puffy. It's not decay or bacteria or something like that. He sees the dentist fairly often, and the dentist only says that if he ever has to have braces, it'll be difficult, but he's not worried*

about it. We tell Morgan that if he gargles he'll get bigger teeth, and that seems a little bit of an incentive to him. I guess he hasn't been teased about it, or if he has, it hasn't bothered him because he hasn't mentioned it.

Of course, the medications suppress a child's immune system, leaving him at increased risk of infection. A young child's immune system is underdeveloped to begin with—that's one reason that even normal children sometimes seem to get sick more than adults. On top of that, active young children like to play in the dirt and to put truly astonishing things into their mouths.

As JoLayna Arndt notes, it's important to be especially vigilant about this in the first months after the transplant. (JoLayna donated part of her liver to her young son, Ashton.) Here she describes some of the precautions she takes:

> We are very careful, and we are probably more strict than most families. His transplant was in November, so we didn't have visitors over to our house until April, and even then we were very careful about who comes. We discourage visitors, especially if they are sick. We attend church weekly, but we don't take him during the winter. We wash him a lot, and I don't put him in grocery carts. I don't take him to the store at all during the winter. We also do lots of hand washing with antibacterial hand soap. Sometimes my hands get very dry, and I asked for advice. I was told that it would be better to just wash my hands under water a hundred times a day rather than using soap 50 times a day. So sometimes I just run my hands under water.

> We don't let him play in the dirt. We do have a sandbox we keep a cover on, and we let him play in the sand, but that's about it. It presents quite a challenge at times because my dad owns a houseboat down at Lake Powell. Ashton can't get in the water there because there's so much bacteria. It's not a healthy lake. He can't shower on the houseboat, so we have to bring fresh water on the houseboat for him, and we use water purification tablets. But I think in a couple of years when he's ready to get in the water and ski we probably will let him.

> We don't let him have fresh fruit unless it's been peeled or cooked. We don't give him anything unpasteurized. We don't let him have meat from fast-food restaurants. No raw eggs. No cookie dough.

> *At first I was really scared and didn't let his sister hold him a lot. But
> now we just make sure she washes her hands. She goes to preschool, and
> we make sure she washes her hands before she touches him, and we make
> sure he doesn't touch any of her papers from preschool. We're normaliz-
> ing a lot more and a lot faster than I thought we would. Sometimes we
> forget he had a transplant.*

In the six years since Morgan's transplant, Mike Browning and his wife have
relaxed many of the strict rules they had established to decrease the chance
of infection. One thing that helped was to give him preventive doses of an
antibiotic during the winter:

> *We rarely took him out of the house, certainly not into enclosed
> spaces, for about six months. So no grocery store, no theater, things like
> that. We limited the number of people who would come over, and they
> couldn't come over if they were sick. Whenever anybody did come over we
> had them do a lot of hand washing. He didn't even get a cold in his first
> year of life.*

> *The only thing we do now is, if there's a child with chickenpox, we
> would keep Morgan out of school until the incubation period was over. He
> can't get the chickenpox vaccine because it's an attenuated, live-virus vac-
> cine, and you can't give a live-virus vaccine to someone who's immuno-
> compromised. He's had colds and flus and we treat him just like any other
> kid. He has had sinus infections. At one point the surgeon did this outpa-
> tient sinus surgery where he cleans out the sinuses, but that didn't really
> eliminate the problem. He started getting sinus infections again, and so
> what we do now is, during the cold season, we use an antibiotic called
> Zithromax. It's a new one that's approved for children and doesn't affect
> the cyclosporine absorption the way some others do. We give him a cou-
> ple of doses each weekend, and that has basically knocked out the sinus
> infections.*

For more on a child's long-term survival after transplant, see Chapter 8, *Anti-
Rejection Drugs*, and Chapter 9, *Living with a Transplant*. There are three
things in particular that parents of transplanted children should keep in
mind.

First, as transplant coordinator Joan Miller notes, children may—or may
not—show some subtle but definite signs of organ rejection:

Unlike adults, children do show some overt symptoms of rejection. A child may lose his appetite. He may have gastrointestinal symptoms. He might get an upset stomach and throw up. He might have diarrhea or a tummy ache. But these are vague, vague symptoms, not any one thing that you can really absolutely put your finger on and say, "This is it."

Keep an eye on such symptoms, but don't assume that their absence means that your child is fine. There's no substitute for regular clinic visits and careful examination of lab work and (often) biopsy results in detecting rejection.

Second, as discussed more fully in Chapter 9, anyone taking a long-term course of immunosuppressive medication is especially at risk for developing cancer, including a disorder called post-transplant lymphoproliferative disorder (PTLD). Children seem to have a higher probability of developing PTLD than do adults.

PTLD is a very serious disorder, and especially if it is not caught early, the prognosis can be grim. Unfortunately, it's not easy to notice the early warning signs of PTLD since its symptoms are quite variable, and can include mild fever, sore throat, and inflammation of the lymph nodes, all of which more frequently are signs of mild infection. While such symptoms might be regarded as trivial in a child who hadn't received a transplant, parents of transplanted children will want to take them seriously.

Finally, though, the best advice one can give the parent of a child who has received a transplant is to revel in their lives and in the renewed health that the new organ brings. As JoLayna Arndt puts it:

I didn't realize how sick he was until he got better. I know it's his age too, but before the transplant he didn't do a lot. I don't know if it was because he was anemic, or because he didn't feel good, or because the liver was enlarged.

He hasn't stopped moving since the transplant.

CHAPTER 13

Living Donors

MANY PEOPLE WHO NEED TRANSPLANTS have the good fortune of being eligible for an organ from a living donor. While most donated organs—about 77 percent in 1998—come from people who have died, living donations are forming a growing proportion of all organ donations. According to U.S. data gathered by the United Network for Organ Sharing (UNOS), in 1988 a total of 10,965 cadaveric organs and 1,824 organs from living donors were recovered. By 1998 the number of cadaveric organs had increased 63 percent to 17,820, while the number of living-donor organs had increased a whopping 225 percent to 4,106.

It used to be that only kidneys could be taken from living donors. In recent years, however, surgeons have learned how to take a part of a person's liver, a single lobe of the lung, and even—in operations that are still experimental—parts of the pancreas and intestines.

It may surprise you to learn that it's even possible for a living person to donate a heart. As described in Chapter 4, *Heart and Lung Transplants*, surgeons used to perform what was known as a "domino operation" for a person with a healthy heart who needed two new lungs. They sometimes found it better to transplant the two lungs and heart into the recipient, after his healthy heart and diseased lungs had been removed. The healthy heart was then transplanted to another recipient. For various reasons this operation is rarely performed these days.

This chapter is intended both for recipients and for potential donors. We will first look at the advantages and disadvantages of living donor transplants. Then we'll see how potential donors are evaluated. We'll discuss living kidney and liver surgery in some detail, and we'll also mention a bit the less common lung, pancreas, and intestine transplants. In this chapter you'll also find two checklists to help potential donors and recipients decide whether participating in a living-donor transplant is the right thing to do.

You will see that living-donor transplants have many advantages to the recipient, to society at large, and yes, even to the donor. Although the disadvantages are significant and are often insurmountable, potential transplant recipients owe it to themselves to find out if they're candidates for living-donor transplants, and to at least consider the possibility.

Advantages of living-donor transplants

There are many advantages to the recipient for receiving an organ from a living donor. The most important is that you're likely to have a much shorter waiting time before the transplant. If you find a suitable living donor, your transplant can take place in just a few weeks—as soon as tests are completed—instead of waiting months or years for a cadaveric organ.

In fact, as mentioned in Chapter 2, *The System*, someone who might be considered only a marginal candidate for a cadaveric transplant and may not even be able to get on the waiting list may be able to get a transplant anyway if he or she can find a living donor.

Living-donor transplants can be scheduled at your (and the donor's) convenience. Do you want to wait a couple of months until after your daughter's graduation? In most cases that won't be a problem. If you're on the list for a cadaveric transplant, on the other hand, you have no choice about when the organ will become available, and if you want a transplant you have to be willing to drop everything and come to the hospital at a moment's notice.

Organs donated from a living donor are almost always much fresher than cadaveric organs. While great strides have been made in preserving cadaveric organs—kidneys can now last more than 36 hours outside the body and still be transplanted successfully—the fresher the organ is, the greater the success rate. With a living donor, the surgeries will take place in adjoining operating rooms, and the organ will spend only minutes outside the body.

Donald C. Dafoe, MD, Director of Adult Kidney and Pancreas Transplant Programs at Stanford University, says:

> *The advantages of living related transplants really need to be emphasized. A lot of people hesitate to ask their relatives, but they really should, because the long-term results are better. The recipients use fewer drugs, there's less rejection, and it's safer.*

UNOS data backs up this assertion. For cadaveric kidney transplants performed since 1990, after four years 66.7 percent of the kidneys and 84.9 percent of the recipients survived. For living-donor kidney transplants, on the other hand, 80.9 percent of the kidneys and 92.4 percent of the recipients survived more than four years.

It's not only the organ recipient who experiences advantages from living-donor transplants. Although the donor has to suffer through surgery and a recovery that can be painful, donors frequently find the experience to be highly rewarding. This can be especially true in the case of a parent donating an organ to a child. As JoLayna Arndt explains, not every parent is given the opportunity to so directly help a dying child:

> From the very beginning we were told, "Your little boy has a terminal illness. The only option is a liver transplant." We were just happy we could do something about it. I compared myself to someone having a child with cancer who is not able to do anything for them. I was well aware of the risks of surgery, but I was hopeful, and it was through prayer that I just knew it was the right thing.

Some potential recipients are very reluctant to ask relatives to consider donating an organ. It is certainly an awfully large favor to ask, one for which true repayment is impossible. There are also other disadvantages, which are detailed in the next section. But Dr. Dafoe points out that both the donor and society as a whole can benefit from living donations:

> My feeling is that you should not take away the opportunity from someone who might want to donate. A secondary consideration is that we have a shortage of available organs. So every kidney that we're able to take from a living related donor frees up a kidney for someone else.

This is true for livers as well, says Emmet B. Keeffe, MD, Director of the Liver Transplant Program at Stanford University:

> By the use of split livers and living related donors, we should really be able to transplant all of the children who need a transplant.

Psychiatrist Larry S. Goldman, MD, of the University of Chicago agrees that it's not just the recipient who benefits:

> One of the things that was pretty clear from the research on living kidney donors is that the people who donated generally had very good feelings about it. Sometimes they didn't feel so good if the recipient had a

bad outcome, if the transplant didn't take or something, but for the most part people who donated kidneys felt very good. They had an increase in their self-esteem, and they felt as if they had done something valuable and altruistic.

Dr. Goldman has himself conducted a study of living liver donors.[1] He describes one of the results of that study this way:

> *In general folks did pretty well, and they felt pretty good about doing the donation. The parents liked the living donor aspect because it allowed them to have more control over when the transplant was done. They didn't have to wait and watch while their kid got sick, and it allowed them to feel as if they were doing something positive and active instead of having the fates make the decision.*

Disadvantages of living-donor transplants

A minority of physicians and ethicists believe that living-donor transplants should never be permitted. After all, you're taking a perfectly healthy person—the healthier the better—and subjecting her to the risks of surgery. Although these risks are quite low in the case of kidney donation, and only slightly higher in the case of liver, lung, pancreas, and intestine donation, they are not zero. Some physicians regard operating on healthy people to be a violation of the initial principle of the Hippocratic Oath: "First, do no harm."

General anesthesia carries a risk. The anesthesia used during surgery kills a tiny percentage of surgical patients all by itself. And any time someone goes under the knife there's a risk of stroke, there's a risk of heart attack, and there's a risk of infection.

These risks are small, but there are other negative consequences of organ donation that are near certainties. Organ donors are certain to suffer some pain and discomfort. Organ donors are certain to lose time from work. This can be considerable—it's not unusual for it to take eight weeks or more to recover from kidney donation.

Living-organ donation not only has the potential for negative physical consequences, it has the potential for emotional ones as well. The great majority of living donors are related to the recipient, either by ties of blood or by ties of affection. The donor is likely to be a parent, a sibling, an adult child, or a spouse. Sometimes more distant family members get involved—uncles and aunts, nieces and nephews, and cousins. On relatively rare occasions unrelated friends, co-workers, or even total strangers volunteer to be organ donors.

Anyone who has been part of a family knows that families are complicated things. People have long memories, and things that happened in the distant past often reverberate to the present. These complex relationships with long histories form the context of any living related organ transplant. It is these complexities that often discourage potential recipients from even asking their relatives to consider a donation.

As Dr. Goldman explains:

> Family dynamics get incredibly messy in terms of deciding who's going to donate, and what it all means to the family. There have been cases reported with kidney transplants where the black sheep of the family was suddenly brought back in and implicitly told that they were going to donate now, and that this was going to be the payback for having been a jerk so many years ago.

Lynn Chabot-Long has written an insightful book about her experience as a kidney donor to her brother Bill.[2] The book is particularly instructive in its descriptions of how the family decided who would be donor after more than a dozen family members and friends volunteered.

Bill's parents were the first to volunteer, but the family decided that they were too old. One of Bill's brothers was the wrong blood type, so he was disqualified immediately. Another brother lived far away and wasn't as good a match as Lynn or her brother Russ.

It came down to the two of them, and Russ insisted that he would do it. He had promised Bill his kidney several years back and he didn't want to go back on that promise. But Russ was clearly terrified at the prospect of surgery—he almost passed out when a recent donor showed him his surgical scar. Lynn wasn't as scared, having experienced the birth of two children, a tonsillectomy, and several other minor operations. Russ also had sole custody of his two daughters, who were afraid they might lose their dad. Lynn finally decided on her own that she would be the donor, and simply informed Russ of her decision, which he accepted.

Lynn's decision ultimately turned out well, but other families may have a great deal of difficulty with this. Some family members may feel compelled to volunteer for one reason or another when they would really rather not. In the next section, on evaluating potential donors, we'll see how the transplant team deals with this situation.

Some families make the decision on the basis of practical considerations. This is what happened when JoLayna Arndt and her husband considered which of them would donate part of a liver to their son:

> My husband and I both have the same blood type, so we were originally both considered good possibilities. We were going to have him go through the testing first, and if he didn't qualify as the donor, I was going to be tested. But we talked to a lot of parents who had been through the same surgery, and we found out what a difficult surgery it was. We talked to someone specifically who had lost twenty or thirty pounds and needed two follow-up surgeries. We changed our minds. We decided that I could miss work a lot easier than he could. It was more of a financial decision for us.

If the decision of a family member to donate an organ is difficult and complex, imagine how much more complex the decision is when it involves an unrelated donor.

For the purposes of organ donation, husbands and wives are considered unrelated because they share no genes. Although they're not related biologically, spouses are uncontroversial living donors because of their ties of affection.

Dr. Goldman points out that it's the donors who are not related to the recipient either by blood or by marriage that cause controversy:

> The other funny thing that we see sometimes is that there are volunteers who are not family members. Now there has been a lot of controversy about whether this is okay. Some people think, "How can anybody possibly donate a kidney for altruistic reasons. There must be some neurotic reason." I think the jury is probably still out on that, but there have been some very successful transplants as a result. You get into trouble depending on the nature of the relationship, and if it's going to continue, and how it plays out.
>
> We've seen people come in who are blatantly psychotic, who say they want to be heart-transplant donors: "I want to die, and here, have my heart." Now, obviously, we're going to turn them down, even though

they're supposedly doing this of their own free will. The more psychological baggage you can see, the more you want to be a little bit careful about doing it.

It's pretty easy for transplant-team members to identify someone who's blatantly psychotic and to turn them down. The difficulty comes in deciding about someone who has no obvious mental illness, but who nevertheless may be donating an organ for the wrong reasons.

According to Kathy L. Coffman, MD, a psychiatrist at St. Vincent Medical Center in Los Angeles, some people decide to donate as a way of atoning for shameful behavior in their past:

> *If we're atoning for something that we've done that's wrong, most of us don't do it by taking a risk that could be life threatening. If you want to make up for a wrong you did, go donate some money someplace, or go do some volunteer work. Most people aren't going to lay down on the operating table and let somebody cut them open, take a part of them out, and give it to somebody else. That's going a little bit above and beyond the call of duty, especially for a stranger.*
>
> *I think we have to bear in mind that even though the risk is low, there is a risk there, and I think that is the crux of the matter when bioethics committees are trying to make decisions about whether someone should be allowed to donate, because there is a risk. It's not an innocuous procedure. Any time you go under anesthesia there are risks of the anesthesia itself, risks of bleeding, surgical mortality, or things that could happen around the time of the surgery—strokes, heart attacks, infections, you name it. I think sometimes we tend to under-estimate the risks involved in these things. It's not the same as atoning through other means. Prospective donors must have a realistic understanding of the risks involved and their own motivation for donation.*

Questions for recipients and donors

The following questions are ones to keep in mind as you read this chapter, as you talk with the transplant team, and as you prepare to discuss living donation with friends and family members. Remember that there are no universal answers to these questions. Every individual must find the answers that are right for himself or herself.

Questions to ask yourself if you're the potential recipient of a living donor transplant:

- Will a living donation decrease my wait time? How critical is that?
- Will a living donation increase my chances of a good outcome?
- Do I have any relatives or friends who might be willing to donate?
- Am I willing to ask these people to consider being donors?
- If not, why not?
- If yes, can I ask for this without placing the slightest hint of obligation or coercion on prospective donors?

Questions to ask yourself if you're a potential living organ donor:

- Do I really want to consider this?
- Why am I considering this?
- Are there other potential donors? If so, how will we make the decision about who amongst us will be the donor?
- Do I expect any kind of payback from the family or the recipient beyond simple gratitude?
- Have the risks been clearly explained to me?
- Do I know how much pain and discomfort I'm in for?
- Do I know how long the recovery period is likely to be? Can I afford that much time off work?
- Am I certain that all my medical bills will be paid for?
- Have I asked the transplant team to refer me to someone who's already donated the same organ, so I can ask detailed questions about the surgery and the recovery?
- If I decide not to donate after first considering it, will I be able to back out gracefully?
- Will I be able to accept it graciously if the organ I donate is eventually rejected? Will I be able to avoid blaming the recipient if that happens?

Evaluating potential donors

The first thing a potential donor has to have is blood type that's the same as—or is at least compatible with—the recipient's. If that condition is satisfied, the potential donor will be put through a battery of tests. Her HLA type will be determined (see Chapter 3, *The Wait*, for more on tissue typing). A perfect match is not required, although the higher the degree of matching, the better. The transplant team will also evaluate the potential donor's physical health. Only if surgery would present the smallest risk will the transplant go forward.

Dave Souza considered two living donors—his brother and his wife—but for various reasons neither was suitable, and he ended up receiving a cadaveric kidney:

> I have a brother who is the same blood type, but he has health problems of his own. He's overweight, he has a heart condition, and he also has really bad asthma. So even though he sought to get a physical to see if he could be a donor, his doctors recommended that he not go through the operation. I was perfectly fine with that because there's a whole different emotional thing with a live donor, too. And my wife was ready to go through the operation too. She just needed to get a blood test to see if she was the right blood type, and she wasn't.

It's worth emphasizing that all of the testing of potential donors as well as the donor's operation are paid for by the recipient's health insurance. The donor pays for nothing, although insurance will not reimburse the donor for lost wages. Some state legislatures, however, are considering enacting laws that would provide wage reimbursement for organ donors.

An interesting case regarding a living kidney donor arose in the San Francisco Bay area in 1998 and 1999. A teenage girl needed her third kidney transplant. Her second transplanted kidney was failing because she failed to take her anti-rejection medications. That kidney had been donated by her father, who was serving a prison sentence. While still incarcerated, he offered to donate his second kidney. This would have left him with no kidneys, and it would have meant dialysis for the rest of his life.

Several ethical objections were raised to this suggestion. For one thing, lifelong dialysis presents many logistical problems for a prison inmate, and the State of California would have had to pay for it. In addition, the girl's kidney was being rejected due to her own actions—she didn't like the side effects of prednisone.

After much discussion, the hospital's bioethics committee ended up turning down the father's request to donate, but not for either of those two reasons.

People on dialysis are subject to a number of significant medical risks, and the committee decided that those risks were simply too great. (The story does have a happy ending. With the girl promising to take her medications religiously from then on, the family located an uncle willing to donate a kidney.)

If there's no health-related reason to keep a person from donating, the transplant team will have a social worker and possibly a psychiatrist evaluate the potential donor's motives and psychological state.

Dr. Coffman explains what she considers when evaluating a potential donor:

> First of all I like to find out, what's the relationship between the donor and the recipient? Is there money being exchanged? That's difficult to pin down. If somebody's got a relative coming from another country, how do you know they're not paying that cousin $20,000 or $30,000 for that kidney? It's hard to know.
>
> The main things I look for are: What kind of relationship is there between the two? Is there any element of coercion going on? Is the donor going to be able to tolerate it if the recipient screws up? Does the prospective donor have drug and alcohol problems himself that are ongoing? You don't want somebody to go into DTs [delirium tremens—a dramatic consequence of alcohol withdrawal], when they're in the hospital donating the kidney. I bring up those issues and talk with them about it and try and find out what the dynamics are between the two. Sometimes I've concluded that even though there may be a sibling willing to donate, that person is not suitable because they've said very clearly, "If my sister screws up, I'll kill her."

Naturally people who wish to donate tend to put their best foot forward when speaking with the social worker or the psychiatrist. This, says Dr. Goldman, was one of the most significant results of his study of liver donors:

> The most important thing that we learned was that prospective donors were presenting themselves and their families in the best possible light so that we wouldn't say no. Several of them gave us misleading or completely fabricated information. There was one married couple that had already separated and were well on their way to divorce, but they never told anybody on the transplant team about it. They sat in my office holding hands and billing and cooing and pretended everything was just

fine. But the minute the surgery was over, and the baby and the donor were out of the woods, they just went ahead with the divorce as if nothing had happened.

In other cases, says Dr. Goldman, people act as if they're happy to be donating when they're actually terrified, or they try to hide family pressure:

One of the cases that we screened was a man who pretended that he was very pleased to be going ahead and doing it, But what actually happened was that after he went through a couple of the tests he finally admitted that he had a terrible experience in surgery when he was a kid, so he didn't want to go ahead with it, and he backed out of donating.

And there were a couple of situations where we felt that there was some subtle or not-so-subtle pressure. Sometimes it happens, for example, that one parent has made the decision to go ahead and donate, but then we run the medical tests and find out it's the wrong blood type, or the liver isn't the right size, or the anatomy is funny. Then all of a sudden there's a lot of pressure on the other parent or another family member who hadn't really been interested in donating, and it's a very difficult situation to say no to.

Many transplant teams have developed a common strategy to smoke out "volunteers" who deep down would really rather not donate an organ. Transplant surgeon Michael Wachs, MD, of the University of Colorado Health Science Center, explains:

As a surgeon I meet with prospective donors separately, and I tell every donor point-blank that there is always some way to come up with an excuse not to do this thing. If the donor feels uncomfortable but they don't feel they can tell their family they don't want to do it, if they're feeling pressured, I can end up being the bad guy and come up with a medical reason why we shouldn't do it. We always make sure the donor has a way to back out.

But although this is a very common technique, used widely in the transplant field, Dr. Coffman isn't convinced that it's always the best way to do things:

I think the problem with these excuses is that they are sometimes very transparent and can cause problems, particularly between friends. It has to be up to the prospective donor what they want told to the recipient, because really it's their relationship. But as a psychiatrist of course I have that leaning to want people to work out their differences, and to understand why something is. A lot of times the recipients are very savvy, and they may have suspicions that the explanation they're being given is not accurate. It sometimes leaves some hard feelings between them.

Dr. Dafoe says that such situations are relatively rare, although it is common for potential donors to experience nervousness and mixed feelings:

The great majority of people convincingly want to do this for their loved one, and there's not that much debate. At some point a social worker closes the door, and when she's alone with the potential donor she says, "We can get you out of this. We know the family may be bringing pressure to bear. We can very gracefully get you out of this." It's normal to have mixed feelings. If they say, "I'm nervous about the surgery," we agree, "That's normal. Of course you would be." And occasionally people get cold feet as the surgery approaches. I've had one or two bolt even the night before. But most follow through in grand style.

Kidney-donor surgery

The surgical procedure to remove a kidney is called a nephrectomy, and there are two varieties: open nephrectomy and laparoscopic nephrectomy. Open nephrectomy is the older and more common procedure. It involves a large incision in the donor's side, a long recovery time, and a good deal of pain. In laparoscopic nephrectomy, on the other hand, surgeons need to make only a few small incisions, recovery time may be much shorter, and there is less pain.

While this brief description may make it seem as if the laparoscopic procedure is the obvious best choice, that's not necessarily so. This section will describe each of the procedures and will provide a basis for deciding between them. It should be noted, however, that to date no carefully controlled scientific studies comparing open and laparoscopic nephrectomy have been published. While uncontrolled studies do seem to show shorter recovery times and less pain for the laparoscopic procedure, that could be because the donors selected for that procedure were the ones most likely to do well. Their experience may not be representative.

No matter which procedure they choose, prospective kidney donors often have one prime question: "Can I get along well with a single kidney? After all, God gave me two. Don't I need both?"

As described more fully in Chapter 6, *Kidney and Pancreas Transplants*, the kidney's main function is to filter waste material from the bloodstream. It makes urine and sends that urine to the bladder for elimination. As it turns out, one healthy kidney can handle this job with ease. Some people are born with only a single kidney, and most of them never even realize it. It's usually noticed only when they happen to get an x-ray for an unrelated condition

After a kidney donation, the remaining kidney may grow slightly larger. Once recovery is complete, there are few if any restrictions or limitations on the donor's activities. Surgeons usually suggest (but don't demand) that donors refrain from occupations that are physically hazardous and from participating in contact sports such as sky diving, tackle football, and motorcycle riding. Such activities increase the chance that the remaining kidney will be damaged in an accident.

If a donor's remaining kidney did become damaged through accident or disease, that would not by itself be fatal. Many people with no kidney function live on dialysis for long periods, and of course a transplant would also be a possibility.

Preliminary tests

If you are still a prospective donor after the list of possible donors has been narrowed down to one or two, the transplant team will conduct two additional tests to determine details of the health and anatomy of your kidneys.

Intravenous pyelography (IVP) is the first. For this test a technician will inject a small amount of a special dye into a vein in your arm. This dye is called a radiopaque dye, because x-rays cannot pass through it. The dye circulates into your kidneys and urinary tract, outlining important structures as x-ray photos are taken. This allows the radiologist to see whether you have any blockages in either of your kidneys. IVP is painless and takes only a few minutes.

The renal arteriogram (also called a renal angiogram) is, unfortunately, a more invasive test that many people find to be unpleasant. The idea this time is to make a detailed map of the blood vessels in your kidneys. Among other things, the doctors want to decide which of your kidneys to take, and they want to know in advance how many blood vessels each of your kidneys have, the exact route they take, and whether they have any blockages.

The arteriogram again involves the injection of a radiopaque dye, but in this case the dye cannot be injected into your arm. Instead, a doctor will insert a catheter (a flexible tube) into a large blood vessel in your groin. She'll then thread that catheter through the artery until it reaches your kidney, where she'll release the dye and take x-ray photos. When the dye is released, many people feel back pain and a sensation of intense heat. Lynn Chabot-Long describes it as feeling like a red-hot poker was being stabbed into her back. Fortunately this sensation lasts for only a few seconds, but it may be repeated several times.

In recent years more and more transplant programs have begun substituting a test called magnetic resonance angiography (MRA) for both IVP and the renal arteriogram. This test involves the painless injection of a non-radioactive dye, and results in a three-dimensional image of the kidney's blood vessels.

Open nephrectomy

On the basis of the preliminary tests, the transplant surgeon will decide which kidney to take. All other things being equal, she'd prefer to take the left kidney, since it has a longer renal vein than the right, making it easier to transplant. In addition, the right kidney usually sits behind the lowest rib, a portion of which sometimes must be removed to gain access. The left kidney, on the other hand, is not behind a rib in most people.

But sometimes there are good reasons to go to the extra trouble of taking the right kidney. In Lynn Chabot-Long's case, for example, the tests revealed that her left kidney had four arteries, while her right kidney had only two. The extra arteries would make both the nephrectomy and the transplant more complicated.

Open nephrectomy is major surgery done under general anesthesia. If your left kidney is to be taken, you'll be placed on your right side on the operating table, and vice versa if the right kidney is to be taken. Once you're completely under, the surgeon will make an incision starting on your side near your lowest rib and continuing forward toward your groin. The incision will typically be nine to twelve inches long. After carefully cutting through underlying muscle, and removing a portion of the lower rib, if necessary, the surgeon will clamp off the kidney's blood vessels and the ureter (which carries urine to the bladder). Then she'll cut the vessels, remove the kidney, and flush it with a cold solution to preserve it until it is transplanted. She'll hand it off to the team working on the recipient, after which the surgical team will slowly sew you back up.

It's a cruel irony of open nephrectomies that the donor generally takes a longer time to heal than the recipient. It's typical for the recipient to be able to hobble down the hall to the donor's room the day after surgery. The donor isn't going to be doing any hobbling for at least a few days. That's because the donor kidney is covered by a good deal of muscle tissue, which must be cut through and then sewn together, and which takes some time to heal. Since the surgeons place the transplanted kidney in the lower abdomen of the recipient, not its natural position (see Chapter 6), there's no need to cut through so much muscle tissue, and the recipient starts moving around more quickly.

Nevertheless, says Dr. Dafoe, the donor is likely to be able to leave the hospital in just a few days:

> For living kidney donors who undergo the open approach, the main thing is pain. It depends on their personality and all that, but if you can get pain under control, then they can go home in three or four days.

But that doesn't mean that the donor is going to be going back to work quickly. After an open nephrectomy, you won't be able to exert yourself very much for at least four to eight weeks.

Laparoscopic nephrectomy

The major advantage of laparoscopic nephrectomy is apparently a much faster recovery time. A laparoscope is an instrument inserted through a small hole in the abdominal cavity. This instrument has an optical system that allows the surgeon to see what's going on. Other surgical instruments—clamps, scissors, and the like—are inserted through several other small holes. Since the surgeon is performing the procedure through a series of small holes, laparoscopic surgery is sometimes called "keyhole" surgery.

Dr. Wachs explains further:

> Laparoscopic nephrectomy is a procedure that's fairly early in its development. I think initially people who are thin and well built and have a preoperative study that shows that we can safely take out the left kidney are the better candidates. The right kidney is a little more difficult to

take out laparoscopically and so that will be reserved until we've gained experience on the left. The left kidney has a much longer renal vein than the right kidney. In the right kidney, it's more difficult to safely transect the vein and be left with enough vein to perform the transplant and at the same time ensure that there's no harm to the donor. Since this is a relatively new procedure, we're being fairly conservative in patient selection and limiting this to left kidneys, but I think that as our experience grows we'll be much more liberal in the use of this. Then anyone who is a candidate to donate will probably be a candidate for laparoscopic nephrectomy.

Just as in open nephrectomies, laparoscopic nephrectomies are done under general anesthesia, and the donor is laid on her right side. The surgeon then makes three or four half-inch incisions below the bottom rib on the left side. Through one of those incisions the surgeon places a small video camera, so the entire operation can be watched on monitors. Through another he'll place a tube through which air is introduced into the belly, blowing it up like a balloon. This gives the camera and the other instruments room to move around. Through the third and sometimes a fourth incision the surgeon places his other instruments.

Once the surgeon frees the kidney from its surrounding connective tissue, he'll cut the blood vessels and the ureter. Then he'll make a two-inch incision just below the belly button. Through that incision he'll insert a high-tech version of a Ziploc plastic bag. The kidney goes into the bag, the bag is sealed, and then the bagged kidney is pulled out.

Dr. Wachs explains the advantages of laparoscopic surgery:

The obvious advantage is that the patients have much smaller incisions. Since we're not going through all the muscles on their side, as we normally do for the open procedure, the recovery is much faster, and there is less pain after surgery. The patient spends an average of one to two days in the hospital as opposed to three to four days for the open procedure. Their need for pain medication is a lot less. With this technique most are off pain medication within a week, whereas with the open technique most patients are on pain medication for up to two to three weeks after the surgery.

The long-term recovery with things like numbness and tingling around the incision or muscle weakness or even a hernia formation is much better with this procedure because it's a smaller incision and it's on the front of the abdominal cavity where it's much easier to heal. Donors who get the laparoscopic procedure feel well enough to go back to work within a couple of weeks, depending on what they do. If they're doing heavy mechanical labor, then it may be a little bit longer. If they're just doing desk work they can go back within a week or two. Some people choose to take more time off, but I think that the recovery is probably about two or three weeks faster.

I think this procedure will eventually supplant the open surgery because the risks don't seem to be a lot higher. The more experience we surgeons get the easier it's going to be, and patients are going to demand to have it done this way because they're going to recognize that it's a less painful and faster recovery.

Although Dr. Wachs is a strong proponent of the laparoscopic procedure, he acknowledges that there are disadvantages, and some surgeons are skeptical. The surgery is a bit more challenging to learn, he says, and it takes a while to get proficient at it. In an open procedure, once the kidney is separated from its blood supply it can be removed fairly quickly and flushed with the pre-servative solution. In laparoscopic surgery, on the other hand, it takes a bit longer to get the kidney out, and some surgeons worry that it can be dam-aged during that process.

Despite these disadvantages, Dr. Wachs expects most of the skeptics to be converted within a few years:

There are still skeptics. I think those are people who are less familiar with laparoscopic surgery to begin with. When you've been doing some-thing successfully for twenty or thirty years, then it's hard to convince them to switch.

I think skepticism is good because right now the most important thing with live donors is that you ensure their safety. You're taking a healthy person who really doesn't get anything out of their donation—other than the fact that they're helping somebody close to them—and you put them through surgery. For the last twenty or thirty years we've developed the open procedure to do that very safely with extremely low risk to the donor. Even though the recovery time was four to six weeks, those people went back to normal life with very low risk. Any time you try to do some-thing new, you have to prove that you can do it just as safely. So there are some skeptics. I, in fact, was very skeptical until we started doing it. I

went to the University of Maryland, where the technique was developed,
to learn how to do this, and then the people from Maryland came out here
to help us do our first couple of cases. After seeing a few of them and
doing a few of them, my skepticism faded.

At this writing, the laparoscopic procedure is being done by only a handful of transplant teams around the country. Unless the recipient is receiving treatment from one of those teams, the donor is not likely to have much of a choice about which procedure to undergo. The number of teams using the laparoscopic technique is likely to increase over the next few years, however.

Liver-donor surgery

Since people have two kidneys but only one liver, some people find it puzzling that a living donor is a possibility for a liver transplant. In fact, the liver is a very large organ with several segments. Surgeons have discovered ways to remove only a single segment. Moreover, liver tissue regenerates. That means that the remaining portion of the donor's liver will—within just a few months—expand to make up the portion that's missing. It also means that the small portion of the liver transplanted into a child, for example, will grow with the child, and will remain completely functional and normal in size (although somewhat unusual in shape) as the child reaches adulthood.

Dr. Wachs explains that living-donor liver transplants grew out of surgeons' experience with cadaveric transplants, and at first was only used if the recipient was a child:

> *What people started doing first was taking whole livers from cadaver*
> *donors and splitting off a small portion of that liver, the left lateral seg-*
> *ment, and transplanting that small portion into a baby. Then, about ten*
> *years ago, somebody decided that if that small portion is enough for a*
> *baby, what we can do is just take that small portion out of a living person*
> *and transplant it into a baby. It was developed for pediatric patients, and*
> *there were some problems at first but over the last ten years, it has*
> *become a very standard procedure for children.*

More recently, says Dr. Wachs, surgeons have developed ways for adults to receive livers from living donors, although different transplant programs have different ways of doing the surgery:

In the last few years, several programs around the world, including our own, have started to do live liver donations for adult recipients. You have to take a much larger portion of the liver for the adult recipient, and the way we've been doing it is by taking the right side of the liver from the adult donor and giving it to the adult recipient. The liver is a unique organ in that it regenerates, so that within about a month or two after transplant, the donor liver has regenerated back to normal size. It doesn't recreate the missing anatomy, it just grows larger. It's still only the left side in the donor and the right side in the recipient.

There are other places in the country who feel that the left side of the liver is the correct portion to take from a living donor to a recipient. There are programs in Japan and in China that are doing variations of what we're doing. They take three-quarters of the liver in Hong Kong. In Japan, they think the left side is useful in some instances and the right side in others. It hasn't been determined yet whether the right side is the way to go or whether the left side is better. Those are technical matters that will be solved eventually, and it may turn out that one's right in one situation and the other's right in another. I think that in the next five years this will become a fairly standard way to get a liver transplant.

On both the donor and the recipient sides, liver transplants are more complex than kidney transplants. Dr. Wachs explains:

For the recipient it's about the same surgery they would go through for a cadaveric organ—in other words, it's a pretty complex surgery. It may even be a little bit more complex because we're dealing with smaller blood vessels to hook up. For the donor, it's a pretty large surgery, and it's complex, but I think it's a safe surgery for a healthy donor. So far our experience has been very good and we haven't had any major problems, and I think that with time the risk to the donor won't be a whole lot more than the risk of living kidney donations. The donor surgery takes about four hours, and the recipient surgery takes four to six hours.

(See Chapter 5, *Liver Transplants*, for more details on the recipient's surgery.)

JoLayna Arndt had a difficult time with her liver donation surgery and its aftermath, but she says she would do it again:

I think it's important for a donor to realize how major a surgery they're getting themselves into. All of us love our children and would do what we could for them, but it's important for parents to understand that a child could reject a parent's liver as easily as a cadaver's. There is no difference nationally in survival rate. It's also important for them to realize that it takes a long period of time for recovery, and that extra help is needed to take care of the child. But I would do it again in an heartbeat because the result has been wonderful for us.

The surgery was really awful. It was an eight-hour surgery for me. I'd had a C-section before so I thought I knew what I was getting myself into, but they told me it's much worse than that. It was very painful, especially after I got home. In the hospital it was okay because there were a lot of drugs. But when I came home the Percoset (a strong, narcotic pain medicine) made me very nauseated, so I just went off pain medication except for Tylenol. The pain went away after a few weeks. It took me about three or four months to regain my energy. I've had problems with my shoulders—my collarbone where it attaches to the rib cage—ever since the surgery. That's close to where they made the incision, and they used rib spreaders. I've been to lots of specialists, but they really can't figure out what is wrong with me, but I didn't have this problem before the surgery and I have it now.

JoLayna's lengthy surgery and protracted recovery period are not typical. In fact, she spent more time on the table than was necessary to remove the liver segment because the surgeons simultaneously working on her son experienced a few delays. Since Ashton had had previous surgeries, he had some scar tissue, which took the surgeons extra time to deal with.

Dr. Keeffe points out that although the donor experiences major surgery, the risks are relatively small, and the recovery period is usually about the same as for kidney donors:

The mortality rate for donors is very low. There have only been a few mortalities. It's well below one percent. For the donor, recovery is generally somewhere between four to eight weeks out of work in terms of getting back on their feet.

It's sometimes not easy to decide whether to go for a living-donor liver transplant or to wait for a cadaveric donor. JoLayna explains that different transplant teams have different preferences in the matter:

From the beginning when we found out that he may have biliary
atresia we were told that a living donation was probably the best option
for him. The wait for a cadaver donor here in Utah is a little bit longer
than some other places. We thought that if a liver comes in time, we'll do
that, and if not we'll go ahead with living donation. My transplant cen-
ter's feeling is, do the transplant before the child gets too sick. I know a lot
of centers will wait for a cadaver liver to come in, and if it doesn't at the
last minute they'll do a living donation. Our center emphasizes the living
donation more than the cadaveric.

Other living-donor surgeries

Although still in their early stages at this writing, some transplant programs
are experimenting with using living donors for lung, pancreas, and intestinal tissue. In each case a small portion of the organ is removed.

The most interesting situation is with living-donor lung transplants. Both
children and adults have been the recipients. Since one donor cannot spare
as much lung tissue as the recipient needs, two donors must be found. Surgeons take the right lower lobe of the lung from one donor, and the left
lower lobe from the other.

The University of Southern California has pioneered this procedure. In a
study of 60 cases involving 120 donors, the one-year survival rate of recipients was 72 percent—about the same as for cadaveric lung transplants.
None of the donors died, although four required additional surgeries to correct problems and ten others suffered significant side effects, most of which
resolved themselves within four months. The average donor experienced a
15 percent decrease in lung function. [3]

One thing to remember about experimental procedures such as these is that
your health-insurance provider may balk at reimbursing you for either the
donor's or the recipient's surgery. If you are given the option of participating
in these procedures, be sure that you are completely clear about who will be
paying for what before making any decisions.

CHAPTER 14

Donors and Recipients

THE EMOTIONAL CONNECTION among the recipient of a transplant, the donor, and the members of their families is far more complex than most people realize. In Chapter 10, *Emotional Responses,* we discussed some of the emotional issues that can arise simply from having a foreign organ in your body. In this chapter, we'll look at the relationship between donors and recipients, and the question of when, whether, and how to make contact.

Some people express surprise at the idea that this is even a question worth considering. If you're not in the situation, it's easy to think, "Why on Earth wouldn't a recipient want to contact the donor's family to express gratitude?" or "When donor families know about the disposition of the organs, it helps them deal with the loss of their loved one." But anyone involved in the situation knows it's not so cut and dried.

In the first part of this chapter, we'll examine some of the nuances of the remarkable connection between donors and recipients. We'll discuss the differing opinions on whether or not contact is a good idea. In general, this chapter is restricted to cadaveric transplants. Living donors are discussed in Chapter 13, *Living Donors.*

As we all know, there are just not enough donors out there. Many transplant recipients choose to become involved in efforts to increase organ donation rates. In the second part of the chapter, we'll look at some of the ethical and political issues in this area, and we'll suggest opportunities for involvement.

Contact

Most transplant teams and organ procurement organizations (OPOs) operate under similar rules when it comes to the issue of contact between recipients and donors: they will not give specific information to donors about recipients or to recipients about donors.

You won't be able to get names and addresses, for example. This is an effort to give both donors and recipients privacy in what for both parties is likely to be an extremely trying and emotional time. The donors have just lost a loved one, in most cases unexpectedly, and they've just made the often wrenching decision to donate their organs. The recipients, on the other hand, have in many cases been suffering serious illness for some time, and then they're subjected to the ordeal of surgery and recovery. For both parties it should be a time to heal, and as we will see, it's not necessarily the best idea for the families to meet, especially in the immediate aftermath of these traumatic events.

On the other hand, most transplant teams and OPOs are willing to provide some level of non-identifying detail. If you're a recipient, you may be able to learn where your organ was procured, and some general details about the donor. If you're a member of a donor family, you may be able to learn how many of your loved one's organs were transplanted, and sometimes how the recipients are doing. Transplant coordinator Joan Miller explains:

> Usually one of the first questions they'll ask is, "Where did my donor come from? Was it a man or a woman? How did they die?" And we'll give them that information, but all we tell them about a donor is age, sex, and cause of death.

Kidney-pancreas recipient Lori Noyes learned a few details about her donor, but she was also concerned with the other recipients:

> All I know about the donor is that he was thirty-two, very close to my age. He was a male, and he died in Lancaster [California]. I could have found out how he died, but it never occurred to me to ask. I went over to the transplant center and said, "May I know how the other recipients are doing? I want to know that they're doing as well as I am." They told me that yes, the recipients were all doing very well. I said, "Oh, I'm so glad."

While OPOs will not give you direct contact information, almost all are willing to convey anonymous letters and messages from donor family to recipient and vice versa. They may even be willing to give you guidelines on what to say in such a letter. Despite their willingness to facilitate this sort of communication between donors and recipients, the OPO will never pressure you to write or respond.

What to write

If you're a recipient and you do choose to write, you could write about your illness and how much you needed the organ, and you could write about how much better you're doing now. You could express your sorrow at the donor family's loss and your gratitude that they were able to think of others at such a devastating time in their lives. You should probably avoid directly expressing the idea that their loved one's death was perhaps for the best, or was God's will, since the result was that you were allowed to live. The donor family is unlikely to agree that your life is worth more than their loved one's, and they will not find that suggestion at all comforting.

If you're a member of a donor family, you could write a bit about your loved one, his likes and dislikes, his hopes and dreams, and you could express your hope that the recipient is feeling better now. You should avoid making any demands of the recipient, or trying to instill in them a feeling of guilt for surviving at another's expense.

When written with sensitivity, such letters can prove to be therapeutic for both parties, even if you never get a response. Lori Noyes' experience is typical:

> *I have heard from the donor's mother. I guess it was his mom who signed the papers to donate, because six months after my transplant I wrote a letter anonymously and she wrote me back anonymously. I've only gotten one letter back, but I received it on my one-year anniversary. That was really touching. I know she knows I'm okay.*

Lung recipient Kathryn M. Flynn writes her donor's family each year, and doesn't find it unusual that she hasn't heard back:

> *I know very little about my donor. I know he was in his early twenties, and that he was African American, and that he was shot in Durham [North Carolina]. I write the family every year through the organ procurement organization on the anniversary of the transplant, but I've not heard back from them. Basically, I say I'm doing very well. In the first letter I said how badly I had been doing before the transplant, and that without their gift I wouldn't be around to be a mother to my child.*
>
> *It doesn't bother me that they haven't answered. I think it's perfectly normal not to answer. I've talked a lot to donor families, and they're glad*

to get the letters, but some just really cannot handle the idea of meeting or even corresponding with the recipients. And I think that's perfectly normal.

It was really hard for me to write the letter, but I just felt that this was somebody's son, and that it might help them deal with what happened to him.

Deciding to meet

Even though the OPO and the transplant team will not intentionally reveal identifying details, in a good many cases donors and recipients can piece together this information. This often happens because organs are transplanted within a restricted geographical area. Sometimes there are news stories about the accident that made the organs available for transplant, and sometimes there are news stories about the recipient of a transplant. It's often easy to put two and two together. Other times, donors and recipients who initially contact each other anonymously make a mutual decision to meet.

Psychiatrist Kathy L. Coffman, MD, describes two cases where recipients learned almost by accident about their donors:

Some of our patients have found out by mistake who their donors were. One gal saw actually a clip on TV about a lung transplant donor, and she was a lung transplant recipient. Because of the rarity of lung transplants at that particular time in history and the fact that they said on TV what hospitals the organs were transplanted at, she knew that was very likely her donor. She was a pretty well put together person, and she said it clarified her thoughts. It didn't bother her particularly.

We had another patient who was very bothered by the fact that her mother tracked down the donor and actually made contact with the donor family. She really was not ready in the first week or two to even confront that possibility, and it was very upsetting to her that her mother did that.

While many recipients feel an intense curiosity about their donors, Dr. Coffman recommends that you think long and hard before seeking to satisfy that curiosity. Once you learn who your donor is, you can't unlearn it:

When a person's trying to think about whether they want this information or whether they don't, it's very similar to the dilemma that people face if they've been adopted. Some people don't care to know who their biological parents are. They just accept that the people who raised them are their parents. Others have a burning desire to know, and they feel somehow their identity is tied up in knowing their origins.

You have to be prepared that if you go looking around in closets you may find skeletons, and they may cause you to have more of a burden than you had already. It's difficult to anticipate the issues that may arise.

Dave and Linda Souza discovered that they learned a little more than they wanted to know about Dave's kidney donor:

Dave: I asked a little bit, and they sounded like they wanted to tell me more, but they told me more than I needed to know, too. I asked the doctor that did the operation about the donor. He said it was a forty-two-year-old white female from somewhere north of Sacramento, who died of a gunshot wound to the head. I kind of cringed when I heard she died of a gunshot wound. I have no idea if it was self-inflicted. I didn't want to ask any more questions. I just wanted to know the donor's sex.

Linda: That's the first question we asked when we got there. And the doctor's reaction was, "Why do you want to know?" And I said, "Because I want to say a prayer for her and her family."

Dave: We've never considered contacting the family. We follow up in our own way, in our own prayers.

You certainly shouldn't feel bad or abnormal if you don't wish to make contact, notes Suzan Best:

Right now I'm not sure I want to know about the donor. It's still kind of fresh. It's only been a month. I think right now I'm going to let it stay where it's at, and perhaps in the future I might change my mind.

Liver recipient Steven W. Rahn didn't feel comfortable with the idea of meeting his donor's family:

I would probably feel different at this point, but at the time the donor's family did want to meet me, but I declined. I was just uncomfortable with the idea of meeting them. What I told the transplant team was, "No, I just don't feel comfortable with the idea of communicating with them," and my wishes were respected. Then, probably four months after I was discharged, the organ procurement organization sponsored a picnic for recipients and their families. I don't know whether the transplant coordinators specifically told the family, or if they just figured I would be there, but I found out that they were there. They saw me, but they didn't approach me.

Psychiatrist Larry S. Goldman would probably support Steven Rahn's decision not to make contact:

I think the first thing is to realize that these are very, very powerful dynamics. This is not such a straightforward piece of business. It isn't like somebody who bought you a cup of coffee. This is somebody who really did something for you, and the result is beating inside of you, so there may be a lot of ramifications. It's probably not a good idea to make this decision very early on. There may be an impulse to act one way or another right after the transplant and say, "Well, of course we should be getting together, since we have so much in common," but you don't really know that, and the feelings about the transplant and the donor may shift over time. Once the two families have gotten together, it's a little hard to undo that.

That was certainly the case for Melanie Horne (we've changed certain details in this story to protect the donor family's privacy):

I actually know quite a bit about my first donor, from whom I got a kidney and pancreas. I didn't seek out the information. About two years after the transplant, I received a letter from the family through the organ procurement organization, the local group here, and I wrote them back. Now I have a couple of pictures of her. She was ten years old, from a big family in Iowa. I know it was a Memorial Day weekend, and they were on their way to Burger King, and a woman who was drunk went through a red light and broadsided them. One of the boys in the family is paralyzed and the father was injured very badly, and Jennifer died. Several of her organs were used. I know the guy who got her right lung. I met the woman who got her left lung, but she didn't survive.

It was really quite something to learn about my donor. When I got the letter, my husband was reading it to me since I don't see very well. As soon as he said her name, the tears started rolling. I guess it was because for two years I had what I thought of as simply a graft and at that moment the graft turned into Jennifer's gift. It may seem like semantics, but it really did change it for me. It became less of a medical procedure and more of a miracle gift, so yes, it was very emotional for me.

Although Melanie is on balance happy to know these details about her donor, she found herself in an uncomfortable situation when her donor's parents began experiencing marital problems. The donor's father called her one day begging her to contact his wife, from whom he had become estranged, in the hope that a reminder of their deceased daughter would help bring them back together. Melanie wisely declined to become involved in this situation, and she has had no contact with the family since.

Dr. Goldman says that it's impossible to tell in advance whether contact will prove to be pleasant or disturbing:

> *I have very mixed feelings about donor families and recipients meeting. There are clearly times when the two families bond together, and really have very good feelings, and it's very helpful to both families. The donor family feels as if they've done something, that the death of a family member was not in vain. On the other hand, there's all kinds of craziness that can come out of it as well. And I think the problem is there is no way to know ahead of time whether you're going to end up with a happy scenario or one that's going to be kind of messy. There's certainly no screening of donor families. When there's no screening, you haven't the faintest idea how stable or unstable these people are, or what they're likely to do.*

Dr. Coffman points out that it's difficult to tell in advance how much information is too much:

> *In general, we have moved over the years to telling the recipients less and less about the donors, because you can't anticipate what will be upsetting to them. It can be something very innocuous that would upset them. Sometimes we have very young donors, and if a patient in their 50s or 60s gets the heart of a 10-year-old child, and they have grandchildren that age, that can be very upsetting. You can't really anticipate what may set off a recipient. Certainly the causes of death can be anything from falling out of a tree to a suicide or a drive-by shooting. For a recipient to find out that kind of information can lead to a lot of problems. Sometimes they do find out things like that, either by looking through their own records or from other transplant patients who may know somebody who rides with the emergency medical service. That creates a lot of work for me to clean up, I can tell you.*

Melanie Horne knows someone who received a very unpleasant letter from the donor's wife:

> I really do believe it is a smart thing to trust the organ procurement agencies to use their experience and judgment. I did hear from one person who had a very bad experience getting in touch with the family. I believe he received a letter and the letter said something to the effect of, "My husband was a God-fearing man, so you'd better be good enough to have that organ in you. You'd better be pure enough to receive this gift." It was full of a lot of religion, and it was very difficult for him because the letter was almost accusatory, as if he weren't good enough to walk in his donor's shoes, let alone have his heart in his chest. It was emotionally damaging.

On the other hand, many donor-recipient contacts are joyful and fulfilling. You may recall the story of little Nicholas Green, a seven-year-old California boy on vacation in Italy with his parents Reg and Maggie. In an apparent case of mistaken identity, bandits shot at their car, hitting Nicholas in the head as he slept. The Green's decision to donate Nicholas's organs made international news. Reg Green, a journalist, has written *The Nicholas Effect: A Boy's Gift to the World* (O'Reilly & Associates, 1999), an enormously moving book about this incident and its aftermath. The title refers to all the wonderful things that happened as a result of this terrible tragedy. For example, Italy's rate of organ donation tripled following Nicholas's death.

The Greens have met all seven people who received Nicholas's organs, and Reg has witnessed firsthand the positive power of contact between donors and recipients. He writes:

> In a tiny village in the north of Italy on a rain-soaked Sunday afternoon, I was asked to lead a discussion of donor families. I agreed with a sinking heart: group therapy is foreign to my nature. . . . In this case, there were about thirty of us, from a dozen families. It was as bad as I'd feared, two or three who wanted to talk, most of the rest sitting in gloomy silence. One young woman, who had lost her husband, struggled through sobs to weigh the good results of donating against the crushing loss. Who better than the rest of us there to commend her, but who better than we to know the futility of saying so? Almost none of them knew who their recipients were: I couldn't tell if they were resigned or resentful or simply didn't care. But there was an air of deep dejection over the discussion.

A few days later, during an Italian television program I was on, one of the other guests, a recipient, said blithely he had no interest in knowing who his donor was. To him that was history. He felt like a new man, his business was doing well, and the illness that had nearly finished him off just a nightmare. To my mind came an image of the impassive faces of those heartsick people, the bare room, the hard chairs, and the rain beating on the windows. It seemed like a different world, but it was just the knife's other edge.

Some recipients, however, do go to extraordinary lengths to find their donor's family—researching newspapers, perhaps, to pinpoint a particular car accident on a certain night. Some then charge ahead; they can't wait to say, "Thank you—you saved my life." Many others are shy, unwilling to do anything that might reawaken memories. So they hold off, making do with the scraps of information they've pieced together, and sometimes never do write or make that call, despite knowing with near certainty that they owe their lives to this someone who is a stranger only in name.

Similarly, many donor families choose not to meet the recipients. Some are in a sort of shock for months or years. Some don't want to do anything until they feel ready to smile again. Others are fearful, worried that they won't like them, afraid they'll like them too much, frightened that they may have to go through their grief all over again if the transplant fails. Still others don't ever feel involved: they see as pure coincidence whatever it was that brought the two families together in what, strictly speaking, can't even be called an encounter. Their attitude is simple: "Let's try to put our own lives together and let them get on with theirs."

The most dramatic meetings of donor families and recipients are on television programs when the two are brought together for the first time. It can be hokey and more like the last act of a soap opera than real life. But I can speak to the power of it also. Before the show the two sides are carefully segregated. Both are nervous as kittens, far more so than usual for people going on television for the first time. They sigh a lot, hold hands with relatives, gaze into space. The meetings themselves, however, are generally a love fest. The hostess gives the build up, the donor family member on stage twists a Kleenex in her hands, the curtain parts, the recipient enters, and both parties forget the world. They hug, cry, stroke,

gaze at each other adoringly. After the show they take innumerable pic-
tures, show each other family photos, swap anecdotes. They are self-
selected, of course—they chose to go on the program—and the first
enthusiasm may not last. But I've seen enough of them now to know they
can be the sort of moment when the earth shakes.

Certainly, knowing Nicholas's recipients has enriched our experience
far beyond anything we would have known. They are now part of our
lives and we of theirs. They are still careful with us, not wanting to stir up
the pain, but we always try to see them if we are anywhere near where
they live and they always seem pleased to see us. It's not like being with
close relatives—we don't know them that well—but they do feel like part
of an extended family. Even from the beginning, however, we never
thought of Nicholas living on through them. These were now their organs
and as Maggie once said, "I wished Nicholas would have lived a long
time. Now I wish the same for his heart."

(We thank Reg Green for his permission to use this lengthy passage here.)

Advocating increased donations

After considering the pros and cons of making contact with your donor family or the recipients, you may decide against contact. This is not an irrevocable decision, of course, and you may find that you feel different a year or two
down the road. Whether or not you choose to make contact, you may wish
to consider becoming involved in various efforts to promote organ donation
and transplants. If you do get involved, as a donor you'll almost certainly
meet some recipients, and if you're a recipient, you'll meet donor families.
Although these are unlikely to be the specific individuals involved in your
case, they can serve as valuable surrogates. If you're a recipient, for example,
you may find it easier to express gratitude to these unrelated families than to
the one that donated the organ living in your body.

Volunteer work with such organizations can prove both valuable and
rewarding. According to UNOS, an average of 13 people in the United States
died every day in 1998 while waiting for transplants. Every year, medical
advances are making more and more people eligible for transplant, yet the
number of donors has grown very slowly for about a decade. Donor families, transplant recipients, and those awaiting transplant are uniquely suited
to bring the message home to people who may never have considered organ

donation before. Heart recipient Jim Gleason finds that publicly advocating increased donation provides an outlet for him to express his gratitude:

> *I feel a desire to reach out and offer thanks for this beautiful gift of life that some anonymous donor family has made possible. Except for occasional blind letters sent to them through the organ procurement organization, this is not really possible, so I find outlets for this desire by using the gift to help support others (participating in local and international transplant support groups, publishing newsletters for when I visit patients awaiting their own transplants in local hospitals, distributing free copies of [my] book to patients and their families around the world, recently as far away as Sydney, Australia!). In a small way this is my outlet for that need to express such deep appreciation.*

(Jim is referring to his book, *A Gift from the Heart*, which is available on the Web in its entirety at *http://transweb.org/people/recips/experien/gleason/*.)

There are many outlets for advocating for increased organ donation. These range from sticking a bumper sticker on your car, to donating money to non-profit organizations, to speaking to civic groups, to sewing a commemorative panel on a quilt, to getting involved in the debate over legislative initiatives intended to increase donation. See the appendix, *Resources*, for a list and description of many advocacy and awareness organizations.

Proposals for increasing donation

While virtually everyone reading this book will agree that it's a good idea to increase the rates of organ donation, it's unclear how to reach that goal. Despite all the publicity surrounding organ transplants, despite the transplant stories of celebrities such as actor Larry Hagman and football player Walter Payton, despite heartwarming transplant-related episodes on television shows such as "Touched By An Angel," despite the US Transplant Games, and despite a US postage stamp (issued in 1998) promoting organ donation, donation rates have remained disappointingly low.

According to some estimates, at least 20,000 deaths a year could result in organ donation. But UNOS statistics show that in 1993 there were only 4,861 cadaveric donors of solid organs. In 1998, that number had grown to 5,791, an increase of only 19 percent. During that same time, the number of people awaiting transplant rose from 33,394 to 64,423, an increase of 93 percent. And this, of course, doesn't even include the many people who could use a transplant but are never put on the waiting list because of listing criteria that are especially stringent, due partly to the scarcity of organs.

Donation rates may have increased only modestly, in part because of decreasing rates of accidents involving drunk drivers and decreasing rates of violent, firearm-related crime. These are laudable trends. As a society, we probably don't want to eliminate all laws against drunk driving or encourage the use of handguns to settle disputes, simply to ensure a steady stream of potential donors.

But what policies would be both ethical and effective in increasing donation rates? Below, we've listed some of the innovative ideas that have been suggested. A few have even been implemented in some localities. Without taking a position on any of these policies, we'll present them, along with some of their pros and cons. It is up to you to decide the most ethical and most effective ways of increasing organ donation, and it's up to you, if you wish, to advocate for your preferred solutions—individually or through some of the organizations mentioned above—to legislators and policymakers.

The main source for this section is an excellent book that contains articles, gathered from many sources, on all of the important ethical issues surrounding organ transplantation. Many of the arguments for and against the proposals discussed below have many subtleties, to which we cannot do justice here. If you're interested in these issues, we urge you to read the articles collected in *The Ethics of Organ Transplants: The Current Debate*, edited by Arthur L. Caplan and Daniel H. Coelho (Prometheus Books, 1998).

Required request

Required request is a policy mandating that hospital workers request organ donations from the family of everyone who has been, or soon may be, declared brain-dead. The idea is that many families never agree to donate simply because they're not asked. By the 1980s, largely because of the writings of bioethicist Arthur L. Caplan, required request became part of the Uniform Anatomical Gift Act, which has been passed in some form in all 50 states and the District of Columbia. Hospitals must have required request plans in effect as a condition of accreditation.[1] Additionally, in 1998, having a required request plan became a condition for all hospitals participating in the Medicare program.

Unfortunately, while the laws may be on the books, and the plans may be written down, they are often ignored. Even today, more than a decade after these laws were passed, donation requests are frequently not made. And these laws have no requirement that the request be made by someone specially trained to do so. A request made badly, at the wrong time or with a lack of sensitivity, is unlikely to result in a donation.

In response to this last problem, The Gift of Life Donor Program—a large organ procurement organization in eastern Pennsylvania—has developed a procedure in which physicians and nurses in participating hospitals are trained *not* to ask families about donation. Instead all potential donors are brought to the attention of a team of specially trained experts who then make the request. At a presentation at the 1999 meeting of the American Society of Transplantation, Howard M. Nathan, director of the program, claimed that organ donations in eastern Pennsylvania have increased 43 percent between 1995 and 1998 as a result of this new policy.

Mandated choice

Most people never fill out organ donor cards. Mandated choice is a plan that would require people to choose whether or not to let their organs be donated in the event of their death. This choice could be made by competent adults at the time they renewed a driver's license or submitted a tax return, for example. Most advocates of mandated choice suggest that people be required to check off one of three boxes—donor, non-donor, or undecided—before the driver's license application or tax return could be accepted.

Advocates of mandated choice point out that more than 50 percent of families approached for donation of a loved one's organs decline, yet surveys suggest that a much higher percentage of people would choose to donate their own organs. Advocates suggest that if the burden of the decision was taken from the families during such an emotional time, more organs would be donated. Additionally, people would be able to make decisions about donating for themselves, in advance, and in a relaxed setting. A mandated choice would also tend to increase awareness about organ donation.[2]

On the other hand, those who argue against mandated choice point out several problems with its implementation. First of all, for mandated choice to work, there would have to be some kind of nationwide system of registration of persons and their organ donation decisions, and this system would have to be immediately available to hospitals and emergency rooms 24 hours a day. Americans have always resisted mandatory registration of their identities, and if even the US Census can't get 100 percent compliance while promising anonymity, what chance does this system have?

Second, it's only an assumption that mandated choice would increase the number of people agreeing to donate their organs. A form of mandated choice has already been tried in Virginia and Texas, where the choice must be made by all licensed drivers. In the first six months of Virginia's program, one million people were asked to declare a preference. Of these, 45 percent registered as non-donors, 24 percent were undecided, and only 31 percent registered as donors.[3] Although that 31 percent represents many people who may otherwise not have signed donor cards, it remains to be seen whether this plan will result in an actual increase in organ donations.

Presumed consent

Presumed consent is the idea that unless a person specifically declares that she does not want her organs donated, upon her death she will be assumed to have consented to donation. People who wish to donate would not have to fill out organ donor cards. Instead, only people who preferred not to donate would have to declare their wishes. Proponents of presumed consent point out that 13 European countries with high donation rates, such as Belgium, use a presumed consent policy. Presumed consent would make donation routine, while respecting the wishes of those who did not wish to donate.[4]

On the other hand, opponents argue that there is no evidence that presumed consent policies are the cause of high donation rates in those countries who have them. They might have high donation rates even without presumed consent policies. Others argue that the term "presumed consent" is a euphemism. What we're really talking about, they say, is a policy of "routine salvage" in which society asserts the right to make this very personal deci sion for every individual, in opposition to the principle of individual autonomy. Also, in any individual case it's quite possibly a mistaken assumption that someone who has not declared a preference would consent to donation if asked. What about someone who doesn't want to donate, but who never gets around to filling out the non-donor card, or who perhaps simply loses the card after filling it out? What about a poorly educated person who may not even realize that he has the opportunity to decline to donate? Can it be right to make ignorance equal consent?[5]

Payment for donation

If families knew they would receive some compensation for donating organs, perhaps they would be more likely to agree to donations. The buying and selling of organs is explicitly prohibited by the 1984 National Organ Transplant Act, but there are some loopholes, and of course, the law can be rewritten.

Proponents of financial incentives argue that the principle of individual autonomy should permit people to dispose of their own body parts in any fashion they choose. Some people also argue that the sale of cadaveric organs is justified in order to save human lives. While many people find the idea that a kidney could be sold to the highest bidder to be highly distasteful partly because this is a situation that would clearly favor the rich, they might find a system of fixed death benefits to be more palatable. As this is being written, the state of Pennsylvania is debating a plan to pay up to $300 in funeral expenses for the deceased when their families agree to a donation. This money would be paid directly to funeral homes to make it seem less of a direct payment for organs. Proponents of such policies say that if the death benefit is relatively modest it wouldn't be unduly coercive, and that the altruistic motivation for organ donation will persist.[6]

Opponents of such plans believe that any payment at all would tend to eliminate altruistic motives for donation. If you receive payment in return for a gift, is it actually a gift at all? Any kind of payment would also tend to reduce the dignity that we accord the bodies of deceased persons. The body of a human being is not merely a piece of meat that we are free to scavenge in return for valuable consideration. Additionally, when a family chooses to donate their loved one's organs they should make the decision on the basis of what the deceased would have wanted, on that person's wishes and values, not their own. On top of that, death benefits would be more coercive to poor families than to others. Families thinking about the death benefit might even be tempted to make treatment decisions while the person was still alive based on whether their family member would be a potential organ donor after death.[7]

Donation required for transplant

Another suggestion is that only people who have previously indicated a willingness to donate their own organs would be eligible for a transplant themselves. This would alleviate the organ shortage two ways. First, only people who were willing to declare themselves to be donors would be placed on the transplant list, keeping the list shorter. Second, the number of available organs would increase, since more people would be motivated to indicate their willingness to donate.[8] But like presumed consent, this policy would also tend to discriminate against those who never got around to indicating their preference and against poorly educated people who would lose the potential for a life-saving transplant simply through ignorance.

CHAPTER 15

Financial Issues

Transplantation is enormously expensive, but on the other hand, human life and good health are priceless. This chapter will discuss the financial issues surrounding transplant. We'll see how healthcare plans typically fund transplantation and what to do if you're not covered or if your plan falls short. Remember that it's not just the transplant itself that is expensive. The annual cost of anti-rejection drugs can be breathtakingly high, and we'll discuss several strategies that might help ease that burden as well.

For more on the financial aspects of transplant, UNOS has prepared a document, available online, that is a source of some of the information in this chapter. You'll find it at: *http://www.unos.org/patients/101_finance.htm*.

The high cost of transplants

As mentioned in Chapter 2, *The System*, even a patient in desperate need of a new organ will not be added to the transplant list unless she can prove she has adequate financial resources, either through a good health plan, personal funds, or a combination of the two. The assessment of a candidate's financial resources is sometimes referred to as the "green screen" or the "wallet biopsy," and to many this requirement seems excessively harsh. Why should an individual be denied a lifesaving operation simply because she can't pay?

This is not the place to discuss the debate over universal healthcare or whether access to healthcare should be considered a right or a privilege. The reality of the current system in the US is that hospitals cannot freely provide the extremely expensive services involved in organ transplantation without some assurance that they're going to be reimbursed. Emmet B. Keeffe, MD, Medical Director of the Liver Transplant Program at Stanford University Medical Center, explains:

We can't do charity transplantation because the hospitals would literally go broke. We have to make sure that patients have health insurance that's going to cover their transplantation because the average cost of transplantation is about $150,000. It's a very expensive procedure. If patients have no health insurance and they have the personal means or other family members who are able to put up the support for that, absolutely we'd go ahead and transplant.

That $150,000 figure includes only the bare cost of hospitalization and doctors' fees for uncomplicated liver-transplant surgery. A more complete list of the costs associated with transplant would include:

- Evaluating and testing the transplant candidate
- Recovering the donor organ
- Transportation to and from the hospital for evaluation and follow-up visits
- The surgeon and other operating-room personnel
- Anesthesia
- Hospital stay before surgery (if necessary) and during recovery
- Follow-up clinic visits
- Laboratory tests
- Food and lodging for family members if the patient is hospitalized far away from home
- Child care
- Physical and occupational therapy and other rehabilitation
- Anti-rejection drugs and other medications

When you include these associated healthcare costs, the total price balloons. Table 15-1, based on figures supplied by UNOS, shows the estimated first-year cost and the estimated annual follow-up cost for the recipient of various transplants. All figures are in 1996 dollars.

Table 15-1. Transplant Costs

Organ	Estimated First-year Cost	Estimated Annual Follow-up Charge
Heart	$253,200	$21,200
Lung	$265,900	$25,100
Heart-Lung	$271,400	$25,100

Table 15-1. Transplant Costs (continued)

Organ	Estimated First-year Cost	Estimated Annual Follow-up Charge
Liver	$314,500	$21,900
Kidney	$116,100	$15,900
Pancreas	$125,800	$16,900
Kidney-Pancreas	$141,300	$16,900

Despite these high expenses, transplantation is cost effective. A single year on kidney dialysis, for example, can cost between $45,000 and $60,000. An insurer paying for a kidney transplant would lose money the first year compared to dialysis, but would come close to breaking even in the second year, and would come out ahead in subsequent years, even factoring in the continuing cost of medication. Similar cost savings can be calculated for other types of transplants.

Managing transplant costs

Every transplant team will include someone who will help you manage the costs of transplant. In many teams this job falls to the social worker, but some teams have a financial person, who may be called a reimbursement or admissions coordinator, who specializes in unraveling the tangled web of transplant funding.

Deborah Anne Mast, the admissions coordinator for the liver transplant team at Stanford University Medical Center, explains what her job entails:

> We work very closely with the transplant families to take the financial strain off the patient. I work with them to get their finances in place, and I try to take care of everything for them so that they can focus on their medical side. Patients should always be aware of their financial status, but the transplant facility should assist with all their health-plan needs for transplant care.

Make sure to bring all the relevant information to your first meeting with the financial person, including the name of your healthcare plan and your account number. And, as Ms. Mast points out, it's important to keep track of any changes in your health plan:

> The important thing for patients to know is that they need to keep their financial person apprised of any changes that they have with their

*health plan. Sometimes you'll have patients who have switched insur-
ance, and they forget to tell you. We try to work very closely with our
patients. If your employer changes your health plan, or if they offer you a
different plan, talk to us before you change. I will actually work with a
patient to choose the best plan that's available for them.*

Health insurance and managed care

Virtually all health insurance plans, health maintenance organizations
(HMOs), and other managed-care organizations now cover transplants, but
the extent of the coverage varies widely. You should check your plan's "Evidence of Coverage" document (the transplant team's financial person can
help with this) to see what your coverage entails.

Traditional insurance plans typically pay about 80 percent of hospital
charges, leaving 20 percent for you to pay, at least until you reach your out-
of-pocket limit. Most of these plans also have a lifetime limit of coverage,
after which they won't pay another cent. This is called the cap, and a transplant patient can easily reach the cap in some policies in no time.

Most health insurance plans also will not reimburse for treatments they consider investigational or experimental. While most solid-organ transplants are
no longer considered experimental, some insurance companies have been
known to brand a procedure experimental—and refuse to pay—long after
the medical community has come to regard the procedure as the normal
standard of care. The transplant team's financial person can help you (by getting your doctors to write letters explaining the current standard of care, for
example) if your insurance company alleges that you're undergoing experimental treatments.

In the past, health insurance plans would reimburse providers as they submitted bills, but now many require providers to obtain advanced authorization for most medical procedures. The transplant team's financial person will
be responsible for submitting these authorization requests.

HMOs and other managed-care organizations work differently than traditional insurance. For one thing, they typically pay 100 percent of the bill,
with the exception that patients may be asked to pay small co-payments,
usually under $10, for each office visit. But HMOs have their disadvantages
as well. They often require you to go through your primary-care physician

before you're permitted to see a specialist, and they also typically require you to be seen by doctors and at hospitals that are part of their system.

Kidney recipient Dave Souza says that his transplant experience with Kaiser Permanente of Northern California, his HMO, was a surprisingly pleasant one:

> You hear pros and cons about HMOs, and a lot of time it's cons by people who don't understand, or who just go to the emergency room, which is an experience at any hospital. Kaiser footed the entire bill for my transplant. It still is footing the entire bill. One pill alone costs $79.50 per pill wholesale, and I take eight of those a day.
>
> It cost $37,000 for just the kidney alone, to get that precious gift. The entire hospital bill for that six days plus all of the side charges was $93,000. And they gave us a list. It had two columns: what the charges were and what Kaiser paid, and it was the same number in each column on all twenty pages.

Many people receive health insurance or HMO coverage as one of their benefits of employment. Unfortunately, advanced heart, kidney, liver, or lung disease often prevents a person from working. We'll discuss Social Security disability in the next section, but for now it's important to mention that when you lose your job you needn't lose your health coverage, and if you have a serious illness it's important to ensure that your coverage does not lapse.

If your company employs 20 or more people, a federal law called the Consolidated Omnibus Budget Reconciliation Act of 1985 (COBRA) requires certain group health plans to extend your coverage by up to 36 months if your benefits would otherwise end. You will have to pay the same monthly premium for this coverage that your employer had been paying, but if you have a serious illness those premiums will almost certainly come to a much smaller amount than your monthly medical bills.

COBRA plans are typically available to anyone who leaves a job voluntarily or involuntarily, unless you were terminated for misconduct. COBRA is also available to anyone whose hours are reduced to below the minimum necessary to maintain benefits, or to people who are considered disabled under Social Security guidelines.

Once you leave your job you have only 60 days to decide whether to continue your policy under COBRA. Be sure not to let this deadline pass without taking action.

Medicare and Medicaid

Medicare and Medicaid are two governmental programs that help millions of Americans pay for medical coverage, including transplants. If you are in need of a transplant, you should investigate your eligibility for these programs, no matter what other health insurance you have. Your transplant team's financial person will be an expert in Medicare and Medicaid eligibility.

Medicaid is funded by each state's government with federal assistance. Some states refer to their programs using the Medicaid name, and others have their own names for the program. California's version of Medicaid is called Medi-Cal, for example.

Medicaid benefits are generally reserved for individuals with low incomes or those who are receiving other forms of governmental assistance, such as Aid to Families with Dependent Children (AFDC) or Supplemental Security Income (SSI). Each state's Medicaid program has different levels of coverage. Some cover the costs of transplant and some don't.

Medicare, on the other hand, is a federal program that covers people in several categories. People over the age of 65 form just one of those categories. Other categories of people eligible for Medicare are people of any age with end-stage renal (kidney) disease and people of any age who qualify for Social Security Disability Income (SSDI).

Medicare includes two parts. Part A is free to eligible members, and covers a percentage of basic hospital care and follow-up treatment. Part B, which is optional, covers additional services such as doctor visits. People enrolled in Part B pay premiums.

Since eligibility for both Medicare and Medicaid can depend on prior enrollment in Social Security's SSI or SSDI programs, you should enroll in these programs, if eligible, as soon as possible. SSI is available to people who are over 65, or blind, or have a disability, and who don't own much or have much income. People who are disabled and unable to do any substantial work may be eligible for SSDI. After receiving SSDI benefits for 24 months, you'll be eligible for Medicare, so it's important to apply for SSDI as soon as you become disabled. For more information about SSI, or SSDI, contact the Social Security Administration at (800) 772-1213 or online at *http://www.ssa. gov/*. For more information about Medicare, contact the Medicare Hotline at (800) 638-6833.

Remember that you needn't be elderly to qualify for Medicare (or Medicaid) benefits. Anyone with end-stage renal disease—which means anyone on dialysis or anyone who needs a kidney transplant—is eligible, as Donald C. Dafoe, MD, Director of Adult Kidney and Pancreas Transplant Programs at Stanford University Medical Center, explains:

> *Medicare pays for kidney transplants, so even the poorest person will get it covered. No one is denied a kidney transplant or a kidney-pancreas transplant based on ability to pay, because we've got the government supporting it.*

Melanie Horne took advantage of both Medicare and Medicaid after her kidney-pancreas transplant. While she's happy she was covered, she notes that participating in such programs can end up being a bureaucratic nightmare:

> *The day I was transplanted I became eligible for Medicare under the End-Stage Renal Disease Act, which covered the kidney part of the kidney-pancreas transplant for three years post-transplant. I can say that Medicare has been nothing but the worst paperwork nightmare of my life. It took them a year to figure out I should have been on Medicare, and so everything had to be re-billed then. And they just finally got around to figuring out that I'm no longer eligible for Medicare, just a couple of months ago. They're still sorting out paperwork and they probably will continue to do so for a very long time.*

> *On the other hand, the Washington State version of Medicaid, which is called the Department of Social and Health Services (DSHS), is kind of a blessing. They pay the premium on the Medicare coverage, and they pick up the 20 percent that Medicare doesn't cover.*

> *Anything that gets billed to DSHS still comes up with a flag that I have Medicare, even though I don't have it any more. So they deny it, and then the bill gets sent to Medicare, and then Medicare denies it, so it gets back to the provider, and the provider has to bill DSHS again with the paper in hand that says Medicare denied it. This happens for every single*

thing I have done, every single blood draw, every single lab report, every single doctor visit, everything. All I can say is I'm really glad I don't work for Medicare. I can't imagine that someone who works for Medicare has a very good day if they're in customer service because considering the complications of all this, I'm sure a lot of people call there simply irate. It's really bizarre.

Like most private insurance plans, Medicare does not cover 100 percent of medical costs. You may be able to purchase a policy from a private insurer that will cover the rest. This is generally referred to as a "Medigap" policy.

Transplant patients fare better than other patients with Medicare when it comes to prescription-drug coverage. While Medicare generally does not pay for prescription drugs, it will pay for three years worth of immunosuppressive medications. Even this is not enough, says Deborah Anne Mast:

> *The other thing with Medicare is that they only cover the immunosuppressant medications after transplant for three years. So what they're assuming is that a patient is going to go out and get another health plan. The problem that I have with this is that there are some patients who are not capable of going back to work after transplant, either because they're over 65 or because they just have some other disability or something else going on. And they're not necessarily going to be eligible for Medi-Cal either. So what you're saying with a Medicare person is, "Okay, we're going to give you a transplant, we're going to let you live for three years, but after that you're on your own."*

As this is being written, two bills are pending in the US Congress that would eliminate the three-year limit. Let's hope that one of those bills passes and is signed into law.

For more on the high cost of immunosuppressive medications and strategies for dealing with this, see the section on "Pharmaceuticals" later in this chapter.

CHAMPUS and the Veterans Administration

Families of active-duty, retired, or deceased military personnel may be eligible for partial coverage for transplants through the Civilian Health and Medical Program of the Uniformed Services (CHAMPUS). You must obtain prior authorization from the CHAMPUS medical director for the costs associated with transplant. This is normally accomplished through a summary of your condition submitted by your physician. If you think you might be eligible for CHAMPUS coverage, be sure to tell the financial person in your transplant team, who will handle the necessary paperwork. For more information about CHAMPUS, call (303) 361-1126.

If you are a veteran of the armed services who became ill while serving, or if you are a veteran who is indigent, you may be eligible to receive treatment at a Veterans Administration Medical Center. The VA also provides some prescription-drug coverage. For more information, contact the nearest VA office.

Other sources of funds

If you don't have adequate insurance, here are a few suggestions for other sources of funds for transplant:

- If you have money saved for a rainy day, that day has come.

- You may be able to withdraw cash from retirement or pension accounts. Some plans will let you withdraw funds without penalty for medical emergencies. However, if it's a tax-deferred fund, such as an Individual Retirement Account (IRA), you may have to pay taxes on any amounts withdrawn. Be sure to check with your tax advisor before proceeding.

- Gain access to the equity in your home by taking out a second mortgage or a reverse mortgage.

- If you have life insurance, you may qualify for accelerated death benefits or a viatical settlement. In an accelerated death benefit the insurance company pays you a percentage of the value of your policy before your death. Viatical settlements are cash lump sums given by investors to terminally ill people in exchange for the death benefits of their life insurance. For more information on these options, see *http://www.viatical-expert.net/*.

- Have your friends or co-workers organize a fund-raiser to help you pay for your treatments. (There's more about this in the next section.)

- Try to interest local newspaper or television reporters in writing or broadcasting stories about your plight.

- Check with your church or any fraternal organizations to which you belong; many of them maintain funds for members to use in emergencies.

Fund-raising

If you find that you need to raise funds, don't wait until you get really sick. Deborah Anne Mast advises:

> Another important thing is to do that fund-raising right away. A lot of patients will wait until they get to the top of the list, or until they start feeling sick, to start to fund-raise. I advise them that if they can't put a little bit of money in the bank every month on their own, then start doing some fund-raising right away.

If you decide that you need to raise funds, you then face the choice of whether to do it yourself (or with a small group of friends), or whether to make use of the services of an organization specifically set up to help people in need of money for medical care.

JoLayna and Bryan Arndt decided to raise funds themselves when they needed extra money for their son's liver transplant. They were fortunate to have help in arranging a fund-raising event. As JoLayna recalls:

> We had insurance and we were still stuck with about $40,000. We had a fund-raiser before the surgery. My husband is a hockey player, although not professionally. He's a referee and he plays, so we had the Utah Grizzlies—a local minor-league hockey team—donate ice time at the skating rink. He skated 1,000 laps, and a lot of corporations around Salt Lake City donated a dollar per lap. We were able to raise the full amount by doing that.

As social worker Mary Burge points out, there are important drawbacks to doing everything by yourself:

> First of all, if you are applying for Medi-Cal, for example, and all of a sudden you have this huge bank account, that can jeopardize your Medi-Cal benefits. Also, it's very demoralizing to go out and try to raise money. For most of these families it's very embarrassing, it's crushing, it's terrible to have a can with your name on it in the A&P. Another reason for not wanting to just put yourself on TV and try to raise money that way is that the public is very fickle. The public would like to donate money to a little freckled girl with pigtails much more than to a homely middle-aged man. Fund-raising organizations can advise them about things that have worked or haven't worked for other people.

There are several organizations that specialize in helping people raise money for organ transplants. Some even provide direct emergency grants for medications and transplant-related expenses. All are non-profit organizations, and you'll find full contact information in the appendix, *Resources*. These organizations include:

- American Kidney Fund
- American Liver Foundation
- Barbara Anne DeBoer Foundation
- Children's Organ Transplant Association
- National Foundation for Transplants
- National Transplant Assistance Fund

Gary McMahan, executive director of the National Foundation for Transplants (NFT), explains why organizations like his are necessary:

> *The National Foundation for Transplants exists primarily because in this country 10 percent of the population does not have adequate health insurance to cover the cost of the transplant, and they also do not qualify for any of the public assistance programs such as Medicaid or Medicare.*

Mr. McMahan points out that one of the major advantages of raising funds through an organization such as his is that it provides certain tax advantages to the people making donations:

> *We are recognized by the Internal Revenue Service as a 501(C)3 organization, which means that we are a tax-exempt not-for-profit organization. Donations which are made through our organization are therefore tax deductible, so it provides the contributors with a tax deduction. Without going through an organization such as ours, an individual could give a patient up to $10,000 directly without getting into gift taxes. That money wouldn't have to be reported as income by that patient, but at the same time the individual giving that gift would not be able to take any kind of deduction. By working through us, on the other hand, it works out as a tax deduction to the individual.*

> *There's also no gift tax, even for donations in excess of $10,000. The only limitation is you're restricted from deducting more than 50 percent of your adjusted gross income as charitable donations, but there are very few people who come anywhere near that threshold of giving.*

Organizations such as NFT help people organize a fund-raising effort, and they receive and manage the funds that are donated. Mr. McMahan points out that unless the preliminary organizational work is done properly, it's unlikely that the fund-raising effort will be successful:

> It's important to establish a local group of volunteers who are willing to put some time and effort into the actual grassroots fund-raising. We try to get that group of individuals organized. If it's not organized then it's just chaos. The patient identifies volunteers for us to work through in a leadership role. There will be a campaign chair or chairs, there will be a campaign treasurer who's collecting the funds, and there will be individuals who will take the lead on different types of fund-raising activities or events.

Mr. McMahan says that, based on his 26 years of experience, he's identified five keys to success in fund-raising:

1. There must be a critical mass of volunteers.

> You can't have two people go out and raise $50,000 unless one of them happens to be Ross Perot. I like to have them start with a good core group of about 15 to 20 volunteers, and to build from that.

2. Those volunteers must be well organized.

> There has to be somebody who is calling the shots. You can't run the group as a pure democracy and take votes: "Okay, everybody in favor of doing a car wash raise your hand." You'll find that no one wants to do a car wash, so it doesn't get done. You have to have somebody who is calling the shots, so we ask that there be an established campaign chair or chairs to direct the volunteers, and to ask people to do specific things. You have to have somebody who can say, "Well, Linda, would you do this? John, would you do this for me?" That requires some leadership.

> The patient is never going to chair his or her own campaign. On occasion, we will let a patient's spouse be involved, but they can only be identified as a co-chair. We have to use an individual outside the family, because the family is too busy and too involved.

3. The volunteers must be motivated.

> They have to realize that they have a stake in the outcome. They have to "keep an eye on the prize." There will be some work involved in

this. There's no way to get around that. But at the same time, with all the things that we do in our lives, this could be very meaningful work.

We frequently hear comments from volunteers who say, "You know, I do a lot of things in my life, but this is especially worthwhile, because I'm actually helping to save a life. And I'm not only helping to save the recipient's life, and helping his family get through this tragic situation, but my efforts will actually make that organ donor's life more meaningful."

4. The volunteers must undertake a variety of fund-raising activities.

You can't just set up a car wash and expect to raise $50,000. You can't do it just by writing a few letters.

Mr. McMahan says there are four basic fund-raising techniques:

— Direct mail or direct ask.

I suggest that people write letters of appeal only to people they know personally, and not to people they do not know. When I go through the mail the first things I read are letters from people I know, and the second things are bills that I know I have to pay. The rest of the mail may get opened or it may not. Go to your Christmas card list. Go to your private address list. Those are the people you're going to want to contact.

— Special events.

This category includes putting donation cans out on the counters of local businesses, doing car washes, setting up golf tournaments and charity auctions, and so on.

— Product sales.

We have access to things like candy, cookbooks, and other items that could then be sold. We usually encourage people to sell things where they're going to get at least 50 percent of the cost back into the campaign. For example, the candy bars we make available through Nestle's retail for a dollar, and they cost us fifty cents apiece. We've developed a cookbook from recipes from transplant patients and their families, and we make that available for $4 a book, and they then try to sell them for between $12 and $15, so that the difference is going into the patient's account.

– Cooperative efforts with local businesses.

We've had situations where gas stations would let a group of volunteers come in and offer full service at the gas pump, and the station may donate a dime or a quarter per gallon to the campaign.

5. Donors must be confident that their money will actually go to the patient's medical expenses.

It can't be looked upon as some kind of scheme or con job. That's where an organization like ours also comes in. We provide some assurances that these funds are not under the control of the patient. They're under our control. In fact, we have very strict guidelines about how the money is used. We tell patients that we can't use the funds that are donated for them for anything that would be interpreted as either income for the patient or an asset for the patient. We can't make mortgage payments. We can't make car payments. We can pay for trips to the doctor's office and things like that. We also can't compensate for lost income if they're not working. What I tell a patient is that we can pay for those new expenses that they would not have had if they hadn't been sick.

As Mary Burge noted, one of the most challenging parts of any fund-raising campaign is publicity. Mr. McMahan agrees, but says that organizations such as his can also be helpful in that respect:

We try to get as much visibility and publicity for the campaign as possible. We try to work with local television stations, but for the most part television stations in larger urban areas aren't going to provide much coverage. Television works so much off the sound bite, so it's hard to develop a story. A TV station in a small market can be tapped for some stories if it's a slow news day.

Newspapers, on the other hand, are very good at developing stories about the patient. One of our staff here will help write press releases for the patients and distribute them to all the different media outlets.

Of course, organizations such as NFT have operating expenses. Mr. McMahan explains that he taps two main sources in running his organization: he receives a small amount of funding from pharmaceutical companies and other organizations, but the majority of his operating expenses come from the donations themselves. To cover administrative expenses, NFT keeps 5 percent of all donations up to $100,000 made in a given patient's name. In addition, NFT keeps the earned interest on the funds that it manages for patients. Other non-profit fund-raising organizations operate in a similar manner.

People seeking funding for transplants should be wary of for-profit fund-raising organizations. Such organizations often take a very high percentage of the donations for themselves.

Many people who find themselves needing funds for a transplant find it highly embarrassing to ask others for help. Mr. McMahan says that it's natural to feel that way, and that his organization can help minimize the embarrassment. On the other hand, it's important for people not to be too ashamed or prideful to seek the assistance that they genuinely need:

> What I tell patients is that I will never ask them to ask anybody for money directly. I say that all they have to do is to identify people who are willing to ask on their behalf. And you have to be willing to accept that this is a bit of an ego squasher. You shouldn't let pride get in your way of letting people do what they really want to do.
>
> I talk extensively about the fact that while we may think that we operate as independents in this life, and while we have our egos, and while we don't want to rely upon others, in essence we rely upon others every day. We rely upon our employers, we rely upon our family, we rely upon our neighbors. It's really false pride to think that we are able to stand up alone and meet every kind of challenge that comes before us. We are here to help each other.

Pharmaceuticals

Even if you have excellent insurance or were able to raise funds for your transplant in other ways, you may be faced with an unpleasant surprise after surgery. Anti-rejection drugs can be extremely expensive, and many health plans don't cover the costs of drugs. As was mentioned earlier, even Medicare, which is excellent about covering all the costs of kidney transplants under its End Stage Renal Disease program, will pay for only three years' worth of immunosuppressive drugs.

The cost of anti-rejection drugs, not to mention all the other drugs post-transplant patients must take, can be sky high. It's not at all unusual for a transplant patient to spend $12,000 to $15,000 on drugs annually, often even more during the first year.

Faced with such huge drug bills, some transplant patients make the very bad decision to cut back on their medication to save a few dollars. This decision is a perfect example of the old saying, "penny wise and pound foolish." If you cut back on anti-rejection drugs, at minimum you risk a rejection episode. As discussed in Chapter 8, *Anti-Rejection Drugs*, even minor rejection episodes are typically treated with high doses of medication, potentially leaving you in a worse financial situation than before. A serious rejection episode can result in the loss of the organ—requiring a re-transplant—or even death.

The high cost of drugs

Why do immunosuppressive drugs cost so much? One reason is that most are fairly new, and US patent law gives the company that originally developed the drug the exclusive permission to market it for seventeen years. For the first ten to twelve years of that period, any new drug will be in clinical trials, leaving about five to seven years for the pharmaceutical company to profit from its invention.

It's extremely expensive to develop drugs. The pharmaceutical industry estimates that each new drug coming to market in the late 1990s cost an average of more than $200 million to develop. Although pills typically cost only pennies to manufacture, pharmaceutical companies charge patients high prices because they need to recoup these research and development costs.

At least that's what the pharmaceutical industry says. Many consumer advocates remain suspicious of the industry's protestations of poverty, noting that the pharmaceutical industry is consistently among the most profitable industries worldwide, and that they often sell their drugs for far lower prices overseas than they do in the US.

The limited period of patent protection does provide some consolation for the weary consumer of drugs. Once the patent runs out, any company can manufacture generic versions of a drug, although generic-drug manufacturers do have to prove to the US Food and Drug Administration that their generic versions are equivalent in activity to the drug's original form. Once generic versions of a drug become available, competition usually drives down the price dramatically. The patents on most current immunosuppressives will run out within the next few years, so there's every reason to hope that the price will come down.

On the other hand, not every drug will have a generic version, even after the patent runs out. If no generic-drug manufacturer steps forward to compete with the original manufacturer, the price tends to stay up.

Another factor that may tend to keep your drug costs up is that new and improved drugs are continually being developed. Your doctor may eventually want to switch you from one of the drugs you're currently taking to a new one at a higher cost. Often the new drugs are more effective or have fewer side effects than the current selections. But often they're much more expensive as well. It's best to be an informed consumer in a situation like this, and to confirm that the new drug really will work out better in your personal calculations of cost versus benefit.

Mail-order pharmacies

There are several national mail-order pharmacies that specialize in the needs of transplant patients. These companies may be able to obtain the drugs you need at a lower cost than your local pharmacy, and since they deal with many transplant patients, they're also more likely to have the items you need in stock at all times. If you have pharmaceutical coverage, these companies will deal directly with your insurance company.

Some of these companies offer other services as well. Stadtlanders, for example, publishes *LifeTimes*, an excellent magazine for transplant patients, which they distribute free to their customers. They also carefully monitor drug interactions, and maintain a social service department that can provide advice and assistance with financial and emotional issues.

Another advantage of the mail-order pharmacies is that many insurance plans offer discounts if you use them.

The four mail-order pharmacies that follow specialize in the needs of transplant recipients (see the appendix for full contact information):

- American Preferred Prescription, Inc.

- Chronimed

- SangStat Medical Corporation

- Stadtlanders Pharmacy

Drug-company subsidies

Several pharmaceutical companies that manufacture drugs used by transplant recipients have special programs in which they provide subsidies to indigent patients. All of these programs have limitations, and all will require proof of financial need.

If you receive your drugs from Stadtlander's Pharmacy, a customer service representative can help you apply for these programs at your request. Otherwise you may apply yourself. Participating companies are listed in the appendix, *Resources*.

State programs

If you are a kidney transplant recipient, you may wish to investigate whether your state is one of the 25 or so that have special programs to assist with the cost of outpatient renal medications. To determine if your state has such a program, contact the National Organization for State Kidney Programs at (800) 733-7345.

Although not specifically directed to transplant patients, some states have pharmaceutical assistance programs that assist people in financial difficulty with the cost of medications. These programs tend to be limited to seniors or to people with disabilities. See the appendix for a listing of these state programs.

The black market

As reported in the *Wall Street Journal*, the high cost of immunosuppressive medication has resulted in a black market for these drugs.[1] Unlike the black market in illicit, mind altering drugs, however, the "dealers" in the anti-rejection drug trade are motivated by altruism and give away their products for free.

There are several sources for the drugs on the black market. Some come from sympathetic doctors and other health professionals. Others somehow come directly from manufacturers. And still others come from transplant patients. When somebody has switched medications, for example, they may be left with a supply of the old pills. Likewise, there may be a substantial supply of medication left over when a patient dies. Some of the medication, however, may be past its expiration date and of uncertain potency.

While the dealers usually have some connection with medical institutions, they are typically not pharmacists. It's a crime to dispense medications without a prescription, and federal regulators in particular frown on anyone who dispenses expired medicines. Some medical institutions, fearing a government crackdown, strongly discourage their employees from participating in the underground. On the other hand, some law-enforcement agencies seem reluctant to go after people participating in the underground distribution of immunosuppressive drugs, questioning the likelihood that a jury would convict anyone whose only motivation was to help the sick.

We do not recommend that you get your medications on the black market, but we recognize that obtaining medications this way is an unfortunate reality for some transplant recipients. If you find yourself unable to pay for immunosuppressive medications and none of the strategies for reducing the cost seem to work, you might want to make gentle inquiries of other patients or members of your transplant team about the underground network. If you take this risk, be careful with whom you deal on this matter, and make sure you inspect any medications you receive from this source very closely. Be wary of medications that are well past their expiration dates or that may not have been stored correctly, and don't accept medications that have become damp or discolored or that have any other obvious signs of damage.

In conclusion

The mountains of bills that start arriving soon after a transplant may be frightening or overwhelming. Heart recipient Jim Gleason says that one piece of advice that worked well for him was to ignore all those bills, at least for a while:

> Early on, someone gave us some good advice. They said, "Don't pay any bills." Sounded good to me. Their point was, don't complicate the healing process with concern about a deluge of incomprehensible bills. In our case this turned out to be good advice because, just when you can least handle such an issue, they did start coming in, and they certainly didn't provide enough detail to make any sense out of them. We filed them—in one big file!
>
> Now, in all honesty, our insurance was comprehensive and did pay most of them directly without any effort on our part, so it isn't as irresponsible as it may sound at first.

But then Jim received a notice from a collection agency:

> *Just recently, six months after being released from the hospital, we got a collection notice—for $40! I couldn't find what that was for, but in the interests of avoiding big problems, for the mere $40, I paid it. Compared to the roughly $500,000 in bills that passed our hands into that big file, this was just too small to get into trouble about, I figured.*
>
> *A couple of days later, we finally faced the inevitable and sorted out the bills and insurance statements to see what we really owed. In summary, it was a pleasant surprise to see that except for our new-year deductibles everything had been covered and paid for—except for that $40 item. Turns out it had been carried outstanding for many months. That bugged me—I didn't mind paying for it, but I did want to understand it.*
>
> *By 2 a.m. I found it—a hospital billing error! Out of all that, the only thing I pay turns out to be their error! We are in the process of clearing that up and getting our $40 back, but it was just so ironic. I have added it to my long list of transplant experiences. May your biggest problem be a $40 billing mix-up and nothing more.*

No doubt we can all agree to say, "Amen," to that!

CHAPTER 16

Traveling for Treatment

IF YOU DON'T LIVE CLOSE to your transplant center, or you choose to be listed at several centers (see Chapter 2, *The System*, for more about multiple listing), you may be faced with the need to travel for transplant.

Most transplant centers want their patients to be no more than three hours away. That typically means three hours door to door, not three hours airport to airport. They want you close so you can get to the hospital in a timely fashion when an organ becomes available.

Once you're listed, it's a good idea to make a couple of dry runs. You'll probably be visiting the hospital periodically for clinic appointments anyway. For one or two of those appointments, make believe that you've just been told that an organ is available and you need to get to the hospital in a hurry. Think about what you'll pack and who will do the driving.

Make your dry runs at several times during the day. You may want to try it during the rush hour to see how long it would take in heavy traffic. You may also want to try it at night. Things look different at night, and you wouldn't want to get lost on the way to the hospital.

Once you've had your transplant, most transplant teams like you to stay close to the hospital for several weeks or months after you've been discharged. During that time, you're under the greatest risk of medical complications, including rejection, and it's best if your transplant team is only a short distance away in the event of trouble.

Travel presents both financial and logistical problems for a transplant patient and his or her family. Fortunately, there are solutions to most of these problems. In this chapter, we'll discuss some of the alternatives for air travel, land travel, and lodging.[1]

If you need to travel for transplant, you should check your health insurance policy, which may cover some travel expenses. Some policies cover airfare but not lodging, others will pay a daily rate to reimburse you for food and lodging but won't pay for airfare, others will pay you for travel on a per-mile basis, and still others won't pay a dime. Also, make sure you know your insurance carrier's policy regarding emergency care when you're outside their service area. This can be a particular concern if you're enrolled in an HMO.

Air travel

If you need to travel by air for transplant-related matters, there are a number of organizations that can help, but some of them have certain restrictions, requiring, for example, that you be able to embark and disembark the plane without the airline's assistance. The best place to start your inquiries is Mercy Medical Airlift's National Patient Air Transport Helpline (NPATH), (800) 296-1217. The following list contains more information:

- Mercy Medical Airlift (MMA) uses fixed-wing aircraft to help financially needy patients get to and from care centers for scheduled appointments, but it does not provide emergency transport. Mercy Medical Airlift can be contacted at (800) 296-1191.

  MMA also coordinates three sectors of charitable air services in the US— the corporate aviation sector, the private aviation sector, and the commercial airline sector:

  - The corporate aviation sector includes 750 corporations who are part of the Corporate Angel Network. Participating companies allow patients to use empty seats on regularly scheduled corporate flights. You need not demonstrate financial hardship to use this service, and there's no limit to the number of trips you may take. Adult patients may travel with a single companion, and children may be accompanied by two parents. Call (914) 328-1313 for more information.

  - The private aviation sector includes 4,500 pilots and 32 volunteer pilot organizations across the US who use their own time and aircraft to fly patients free of charge to care centers. These groups are part of the Air Care Alliance. Call (888) 662-6794 for more information.

  - In the past, some commercial airlines have occasionally offered special fares or even free tickets for people who must travel for medical care. Unfortunately, such programs are becoming increasingly rare. Many frequent-flyer programs, however, allow members to donate miles to be used by people in need of travel assistance for medical care. It's best to work through MMA when pursuing this option.

- AirLifeLine transports ambulatory patients—including at the time of transplant and for follow-up visits—up to 700 miles. The service uses private pilots and their airplanes. Although the service is free of charge, you must be able to document your medical and financial need. For more information, call (800) 446-1231.

- Angel Flight provides free air transportation on private aircraft for people in financial need and for organ banks, tissue banks, and blood banks. For more information, call (310) 398-6123.

- The American Red Cross will assist military personnel only with emergency travel and communication. To find the chapter nearest to you or your destination, call (202) 728-6401.

- The Mission Air Transportation Network uses corporate, government, and commercial aircraft to fly Canadians who cannot afford air travel and need medical care. Call (416) 222-6335.

- The Mission Aviation Fellowship supports air ambulance services in 57 countries around the world. Call (909) 794-1151.

Ground transportation

If you have cancer, some local offices of the American Cancer Society have networks of volunteers who will drive you to your treatment center. You can find a list of local ACS offices at *http://www.cancer.org/bottomdivisions.html* or by phoning (800) ACS-2345.

The Travelers Aid Society provides emergency travel and lodging for people in great financial need. Check the local phone book for contact information.

Lodging

Once you get to the city where you'll be receiving treatment, you'll face the problem of finding a place to stay. Often you'll be receiving treatment as an out-patient, perhaps for an extended period before and after your transplant, and unless you're wealthy, four-star hotels are probably out of the question. It would be nice to find a place near the hospital where you and your family could stay at little or no cost, preferably one with kitchen and laundry facilities. Fortunately, there are a number of possibilities:

- If you have cancer, the American Cancer Society maintains Hope Lodges in many major cities that provide free housing on a first-come, first-serve basis for people being treated for cancer and their families. Hope Lodges have kitchen and laundry facilities. For information, phone (800) ACS-2345.

- The National Association of Hospital Hospitality Houses maintains a list of facilities set up to provide free or low-cost housing to patients being treated at nearby hospitals or their families. The houses range in size from six to sixty-four rooms and typically have a common living area. Most have kitchens and laundry facilities as well. For information, phone (800) 542-9730.

- The Ronald McDonald Houses sponsored by the McDonald's Corporation offer lodging to children and their families traveling for medical care. You may need to demonstrate financial hardship to be permitted to stay at some facilities. Others charge a nominal fee of $10 per night, which may be waived if you can demonstrate financial hardship. For information, phone (312) 836-7100.

- Some major medical centers maintain low-cost apartments that they make available to transplant patients and their families who are awaiting a transplant or recuperating. Check with the transplant team's social worker for more information.

- Many hospitals make individual arrangements with nearby hotels for reduced rates for the families of patients. The social worker can provide you with more information about this as well.

CHAPTER 17

The Future of Transplantation

ALTHOUGH ORGAN TRANSPLANTATION is not the front-page news it was in the 1960s, and although thousands of people each year receive transplants, this does not mean that transplantation is so routine that further medical advances are impossible. Scientists and clinicians are hard at work finding new and better ways to serve the needs of the transplant community.

This chapter will discuss some of the newest developments at the time of its writing. A few of these will likely come into wide use in the near future. This category includes some of the new anti-rejection strategies and the ability to transplant organs and tissues that haven't previously been attempted. Other developments, including some promising alternatives to transplant, are a bit more iffy, and are likely to come into use no sooner than five to ten years from now. Finally, there are a few developments, such as transplants from animals and the creation of artificial organs, that are at least ten to thirty years away.

New anti-rejection strategies

As discussed in Chapter 3, *The Wait*, some people awaiting transplant have antibodies circulating in their bloodstream as a result of a pregnancy, a blood transfusion, or a previous transplant. This can result in a positive cross-match to a potential donor organ such that the organ would be rejected very quickly, despite immunosuppressive medication. To test for this, a recipient's blood is checked against a panel of antigens. This test is called percent reactive antibody (PRA), and it represents the percentage of the population to which a recipient is likely to have a positive crossmatch. Someone with a PRA of 50, for example, is likely to be sensitized to organs from 50 percent of the population.

In an attempt to overcome this, some researchers are experimenting with a technique called high PRA rescue. The idea is to remove the reactive antibodies from the candidate's bloodstream before transplant. To do this they use "plasmapheresis" in combination with some immunosuppressive medications. In plasmapheresis, the candidates spend two hours connected to a machine that removes their blood and separates the red and white blood cells from the liquid serum, the part that contains the antibodies. The blood cells are then returned to the candidates along with a protein solution that mimics the discarded serum.

In an experiment led by Eugene Schweitzer, MD, at the University of Maryland, eight kidney transplant candidates with high PRAs underwent plasmapheresis six times over a two-week period. They also received Prograf, CellCept, and intravenous immunoglobulin (IVIG) in advance of their transplants to prevent the antibodies from returning.

The technique removed reactive antibodies in six of the eight candidates, and all six received successful kidney transplants soon thereafter.

Although the idea of using plasmapheresis is not a new one, previous results have been somewhat disappointing. In a news release from the University of Maryland describing the results, Dr. Schweitzer attributes his success to the combination of plasmapheresis and the three immunosuppressive medications.

IVIG alone is the subject of great interest among researchers, since it holds the promise of preventing rejection in particularly difficult cases. Immunoglobulins are antibodies derived from blood plasma that can supplement the body's natural defenses. In the case of transplants, the IVIG antibodies seem to attack the "bad" antibodies that would tend to cause rejection.

Another area of great interest is called tolerance induction, and it involves efforts to prevent the recipient's body from regarding the transplanted organ as foreign. Current research involves injecting the recipient's thymus gland with some of the donor's bone marrow at the same time the organ is transplanted. The thymus is where the body's T cells are educated to distinguish a person's own cells from foreign cells. The idea is to fool the recipient's T cells into regarding the donor bone marrow as self rather than non-self.

New organs for transplant

As reported in *The New York Times*, surgeons are beginning to attempt the transplant of organs that were never previously considered.[1]

A surgeon in Germany, for example, has recently had some success in transplanting knees into four patients. Typically the recipients are people who have lost a knee to accident or disease. Without a knee transplant, some of those patients would have to have their lower legs amputated. In other cases, they would have to walk without the benefit of a movable knee joint. While those four patients have regained varying degrees of movement, a fifth patient was not so lucky. In this case, the recipient had suffered two severe infections after operations to reconstruct her own knee. Although her physicians believed that they had those infections under control before attempting the transplant, the infection returned, and she lost the transplant soon after she began taking immunosuppressive medications.

Other surgeons have had good results in transplanting the trachea, the tube through which air passes from the mouth and nose down the throat to the lungs. Sometimes children are born with missing or malformed tracheas, and other times the trachea can become damaged in accidents or as the result of surgery. Although trachea transplants have been performed in Germany since 1979, only in recent years have surgeons in the US attempted the operation.

One nice thing about trachea transplants is that recipients don't need to take immunosuppressive medication. The trachea is made of cartilage, which does not need to be transplanted with its blood supply, and donor tracheas can be treated with chemicals to destroy any antigens that might trigger an immune response.

Surgeons have also attempted—with mostly disappointing results, so far—to transplant the thymus gland in an attempt to treat AIDS, a disease that attacks this organ (among others).

Some researchers are searching for an alternative to pancreas transplants for people with Type I (juvenile onset) diabetes. In the normal pancreas, insulin is produced by clusters of cells called the islets of Langerhans. Instead of transplanting an entire pancreas, it might be possible to transplant just the islet cells. For several decades, physicians have experimented with islet-cell transplants, but success has been hampered by the fact that the recipient tends to mount an especially vigorous immune response to islet cells. Islet-cell transplants could become routine if the they could be encapsulated in a porous tube that would let out the insulin produced within, but would prevent detection by the recipient's immune system.[2]

Researchers have successfully implanted encapsulated islet cells into mice, where implants containing just 500 islets have reversed diabetes. But success with this strategy is going to be far more challenging in humans. It's estimated that a human would require 700,000 islets. While technicians were able to handpick the islets used in the mouse experiments, that clearly would be impractical with the much larger number required for humans, so some automated system will have to be devised. In addition, the mouse implants were small enough so that the islets did not require their own blood supply. This is unlikely to be the case in the much larger implants in humans.

We can expect the list of transplanted organs to continue to grow, and to continue to generate controversy. A plastic surgeon in Italy, for example, has recently applied to authorities for permission to perform three penis transplants. The intended recipients of two of these transplants are genetic women who wish to have sex-change operations to become men. The third is a person who is a genetic man, had his own penis removed in a sex-change operation to become a woman, and who has now decided to become a man once again.

Alternatives to transplant

Since so many people die while awaiting transplant, physicians are searching for ways to allow their patients to survive longer. For people who need heart transplants, inventors have developed mechanical devices intended to replace all or some of the heart's functions. For more on this, see the section "Mechanical organs" later in the chapter.

People who have experienced kidney failure can survive on dialysis for long periods, and people with diabetes can survive by injecting insulin. There is no comparable way to maintain someone with liver disease, even for short periods. As mentioned in Chapter 5, *Liver Transplants*, the liver is responsible for removing toxins from the blood and also for producing thousands of vital enzymes.

As a way of keeping people with liver disease alive long enough to receive a transplant, researchers are developing several versions of an extracorporeal liver assist device (ELAD) that would be used in much the same way that a kidney dialysis machine is used for people with kidney failure. The ELAD is connected to the patient's bloodstream, where it first removes blood and separates the plasma from the red and white cells. The plasma is then passed through a cartridge that contains either human liver cells or pig liver cells. This detoxifies the plasma, which, together with the blood cells, is returned to the patient. While the ELAD does show some promise, in its current form it's intended only to allow patients in acute liver failure to survive for a maximum of ten days while waiting for an organ.

Other researchers are developing a similar device using kidney cells that could provide an improvement over standard kidney dialysis. While standard dialysis machines are effective at removing waste products from the blood, they can't replace some of the kidney's other functions, which include the production of vital hormones. The "bioartificial kidney," as the device is called, has so far only been tested on dogs, but its developers hope to begin testing it on humans soon. The ultimate goal is to develop a version of the device that can be implanted into a person instead of using an actual human organ.

Xenotransplantation

If there are not enough human organs available for everyone who needs a transplant, perhaps animal organs could provide a substitute. This has been a dream of transplant surgeons since at least 1963, when surgeon Keith Reemstma, MD, of the Columbia University College of Physicians and Surgeons attempted the first chimpanzee-to-human kidney transplants.[3]

When organs are transplanted between species, it's called xenotransplantation, from the Greek word *xenos*, which means "stranger."

To date, despite a number of attempts at transplanting several different organs and tissues from several different animals to human beings, xenotransplantation has not been successful. In addition, there are both practical and ethical barriers to its success.

For one thing, we know that the human immune system is all too efficient in recognizing organs from other human beings as foreign and rejecting them. It's even better at recognizing organs from other animals as foreign. Despite modern immunosuppressive medications, all attempts at xenotransplantation to date have resulted in rapid and complete rejection of the transplanted organ. This happens whether the animal of origin is a relatively distant relative of humans, such as a pig, or a closer relative such as a monkey or an ape. (Transplants from baboons, chimpanzees, and other primates have been attempted.)

Some researchers, including a few working at for-profit companies, are trying several strategies to overcome this barrier. The strategy that's getting the most attention involves creating a strain of pigs that are genetic hybrids, possessing a small number of human genes. The hope is that if the genes for the proper HLA antigens could be inserted into pigs, then the human immune system would not recognize organs from these pigs as foreign and would not mount an immune response against them. (See Chapter 3 for more on HLA antigens.)

Even if the practical barriers are overcome, however, there would still be at least two significant ethical barriers to xenotransplantation. For one thing, animal-rights activists oppose the use of animals for xenotransplantation just as they oppose their use for scientific experimentation. They maintain that we have no right to exploit animals for this purpose. This argument tends to fall on deaf ears to a large majority of the population. Most of us have benefited not only from medical advances brought about by animal research, but also from the nutrition provided by exploiting animals for their meat. To be consistent, anyone who opposes the use of animals for xenotransplantation because of animal-rights concerns should also oppose all use of animals for food, for clothing, and for medical research. The more moderate animal-rights activists would support the use of "lower" animals, such as pigs, for transplantation, but would oppose the use of primates, which are more closely related to humans.

The second ethical objection to xenotransplantation is far more likely to derail research in this direction. It comes from the chance that the practice of xenotransplantation could introduce a new and deadly disease into the human population. This is not as farfetched as it may at first seem. It's thought, for example, that the AIDS virus originated in primates and was somehow passed to the human population (although not by transplantation). In fact, many animals are known to harbor viruses whose pathogenicity in humans is unknown. Who knows (goes the argument) what other deadly diseases may be lurking silently in baboons or pigs, only to spread throughout the human population if their organs were transplanted? It would be tragic indeed if a transplant meant to save one individual human resulted in the introduction of a serious disease into the human population.

Does the desire to save the relatively small number of people who could benefit from xenotransplants justify such a risk to all of humanity?

There may be a way around this objection, though. If it were possible to raise animals for transplantation in a special, pathogen-free environment, concerns about the transmission of new diseases might be allayed. On the other hand, retroviruses like HIV, which causes AIDS, insert themselves directly into the DNA. The most pristine environment could not prevent transmission of such viruses.

Because of the practical and ethical barriers, most observers of the transplant scene remain skeptical—but still cautiously optimistic—about the potential for xenotransplantation. Surgeon Donald C. Dafoe, MD, is probably speaking for many when he says:

> I think a small group of very good investigators should be funded, and they should go about it very carefully and cautiously with the appropriate follow-up and vigilance. What I'm afraid will happen—and there is a profit motive here for whatever company punches this through—is that the cat will just be out of the bag and there will be no stopping it. Then, five years down the road, we may find some horrible consequence. But in general I think the fears are probably overdone, and it should go forward.

Mechanical organs

Since the heart is basically a pump, physicians have long dreamed of replacing a failing heart with a mechanical device. Although there is a 30-year-plus history of attempts to build a total artificial heart, complete success has been elusive.[4]

The heart has four pumping chambers: two atria and two ventricles. The atria are smaller and weaker than the ventricles. The sequence of events in blood circulation goes like this: the left atrium receives oxygenated blood from the lungs and pushes it into the left ventricle; the left ventricle pumps that blood through the arteries to the rest of the body; that blood circulates through the body, giving up its oxygen to all the body's tissues; the deoxygenated blood returns through the veins to the right atrium; the right atrium pushes that blood to the right ventricle; and the right ventricle, in turn, pumps that blood to the lungs, where it becomes oxygenated once more.

It seems as if it would be fairly simple to design a mechanical device that would do the same thing, but there are significant obstacles to success. First of all, it's not just water that's being pumped. Blood is a highly complex, salty fluid, and it contains billions of living cells. It turns out that it's not easy to design a pump—and all its associated valves—that would treat blood cells gently. Most simple designs would result in the wholesale destruction of blood cells. In addition, blood has an annoying propensity to form clots on any surface that's even slightly irregular. If one of these clots broke loose and blocked a vital blood vessel in the lung or the brain, death would follow rapidly.

The artificial heart would have to be made of a sophisticated biocompatible material so the body would not reject it. In addition, it would have to be small enough to fit entirely within the chest cavity. But how would you power it? A mechanical device like this uses a fair amount of energy, so the tiny, long-lasting batteries used (for example) in cardiac pacemakers would not be adequate. And of course you wouldn't want to have to open the chest every few days to put in replacement batteries. The most common solution to this problem among the artificial hearts in use today is to use an external power supply. But that keeps the patient tethered to an unwieldy device that must go everywhere she goes. In addition, that device would have to have tubes or wires that penetrate the chest wall, and that presents a very high risk for infection.

Despite these obstacles, there are several models of total artificial hearts in use today, with more under development. In addition, cardiologists are making increasing use of partial artificial hearts. These are called left ventricular assist devices (LVADs). Instead of replacing the full function of the heart, the LVAD merely boosts the left ventricle's pumping action. Neither the total artificial hearts nor the LVADs in use today are seen as replacements for failing hearts. Instead, both total artificial hearts and LVADs are typically regarded as bridges to transplant. They help people in heart failure survive until a transplant becomes available. However, these devices are expensive and are not used as widely as they could be.

Cardiologist Randall Vagelos, MD, believes that more widespread use of the LVAD could be beneficial, although he notes that if this were ever to happen the medical system would have to come to grips with significant social and economic issues:

> I think if the cost comes down and the risks and complications come
> down it might be a way to dramatically expand the ability to support

patients with end-stage heart disease. There are between three and four thousand heart transplants done in the world every year, total. That number has not increased in the last ten years and probably won't unless some other source of donor organs arises. Considering that there are 400,000 new cases of heart failure in our country alone annually, it is clear that the current options for treatment of end-stage heart failure are insufficient. Whether these devices will become safe enough, and then whether our society is interested in investing in these devices, are huge economic and social issues. You might say that since a good percentage of all the people who die in this country die from heart disease, everyone should be entitled to the possible life-extending attributes of mechanical cardiac support. On the other hand, I'm not sure that anyone is interested in really thinking that globally in terms of expanding our life span.

Dr. Vagelos is finding that in practice LVADs are not always used as bridges to transplant:

LVADs have already become an end point or "destination therapy" for patients. They're not uniformly used that way, but there are patients who don't improve enough or aren't robust enough after LVAD placements to be considered actual transplant candidates, so they are maintained on an LVAD. We have a patient who barely survived LVAD placement because he had lung disease that was more profound than we had anticipated before the operation. We now think that he would not survive heart transplantation. LVAD will be an end point for him. On the other hand, there are patients who have been placed on LVAD in whom there has been a recovery of heart muscle function which was not anticipated, and in whom LVADs have then been removed. In those patients, they've been not so much a bridge to transplant as a bridge to recovery.

Tissue engineering

Many of the problems inherent in mechanical organs—biocompatibility issues, the lack of a power supply, and so on—could be solved if scientists could make artificial organs out of living cells. Some scientists dream of injecting special growth factors into an organ that needs regeneration. These growth factors would encourage the patient's own cells to come to the rescue and regenerate the diseased or damaged organ.

Other scientists dream of assembling a human heart or a human liver (for example) in the laboratory—and eventually, perhaps, in a factory—providing an unlimited supply of organs for transplant.

"Tissue engineering" is the name given to this field of endeavor, and success with complex organs is many years in the future.[5] You can't just take a human heart cell, let it grow and divide in a Petri dish, and expect that eventually you'll have a full-sized, beating heart, with all its blood vessels and chambers and valves. What you would actually get if you grew heart cells in a Petri dish would be a disorganized lump of muscle cells, each marching to its own drummer.

One strategy being pursued is to start off by constructing a three-dimensional scaffold with a special biodegradable polymer in the shape of an organ. In the laboratory, the scaffold would be seeded with the proper cells, most likely cells that were the embryonic progenitors of cells in the mature organ. The cells and its scaffolding would then be placed in the recipient's body, where they would grow into the shape and assume the function of the natural organ.

This is already being tried on a limited scale with cartilage, a simple tissue that does not require a blood supply. Researchers have been successful in growing cartilage in the shape of the human nose and the human ear, for example, in the hope of providing people who have lost those structures at least some improvement in their appearance.

A great many advances would have to be made before more complex organs could be constructed. For one thing, scientists would have to figure out how to get blood vessels to grow into the artificial organ. For another, they'd have to figure out how to get the embryonic progenitor cells to differentiate into all the dozens of specialized cells within a mature organ.

There are also ethical and social barriers to progress in the area of tissue engineering. Many schemes for constructing new organs depend on using embryonic stem cells. But when these are human stem cells, they derive from very young human embryos grown in the laboratory. Since such embryos could potentially develop into a human being if they were implanted into a woman's uterus, some people object to their use for research.

In 1994, the National Institutes of Health convened a panel of ethicists and researchers to examine this question. The panel concluded that the use of human embryonic stem cells for research was ethically justifiable. Nevertheless, the US Congress has prohibited the use of federal funds for this research, although some private corporations are funding stem-cell research on their own. If you believe—as do many in the transplant community—that research on embryonic stem cells is crucial to the eventual solution of the organ shortage, we urge you to write your senators and representatives.

Resources

Organizations

Advocacy and awareness

The source for much of the following material is the Frequently Asked Questions (FAQ) document from the TRNSPLNT mailing list, compiled by Michael Holloway. The list of organizations below is by no means exhaustive. There are literally dozens of small organizations devoted to organ donation.

Coalition on Donation
1100 Boulders Parkway
Suite 500
Richmond, VA 23225-8770
(804) 330-8620
(804) 323-7343 (fax)
coalition@unos.org
http://www.shareyourlife.org/

A not for profit alliance of local coalitions and national organizations who have joined forces to promote organ and tissue donation.

The Gift of Life Trust Fund
PO Box 8703
Columbia, SC 29202
http://www.giftoflife-sc.org/

Established by the General Assembly of the State of South Carolina to promote and encourage organ and tissue donation, to educate the citizens of South Carolina on the need for and acceptance of organ and tissue donation, and to assist with the needs of transplant recipients in South Carolina.

The James Redford Institute for Transplant Awareness
PMB 214
10573 West Pico Boulevard
Los Angeles, CA 90064-2348
http://www.jrifilms.org/

A nonprofit organization devoted to educating the public about the importance of organ and tissue donation as part of an ongoing public awareness campaign. Screen-writer James Redford (son of actor Robert Redford) established JRI after his success-ful liver transplant. JRI has produced several films to promote transplants, including "Flow," which speaks to teenagers in their language.

National Donor Family Council
30 East 33rd Street
Suite 1100
New York, NY 10016
(800) 622-9010 or (212) 889-2210
donorfamily@kidney.org
http://www.kidney.org/recips/donor/

The mission of the National Donor Family Council is to enhance the sensitivity and effectiveness of the organ and tissue procurement process, provide opportunities for families to grieve and grow, and to utilize the unique perspective and experiences of these families to increase organ and tissue donation. Among the Council's many interesting programs, one of the most moving is the National Donor Family Quilt. Since January of 1995, more than 800 families have contributed quilt squares commemorating the lives of those who have given the gift of life through organ and/or tissue donation.

National Organ Donor Sabbath
Mary Ganikos
US Department of Health and Human Services
Health Resources and Services Administration
(301) 443-7577
http://www.organdonor.gov

The National Organ Donor Sabbath is an annual event organized by the Division of Transplantation of the US Health Resources and Services Administration. During the second weekend before Thanksgiving, religious communities around the nation unite to promote organ donation with a wide variety of special events.

Nicholas Green Foundation
PO Box 937
Bodega Bay, CA 94293
(707) 875-2263
http://www.greenfoundation.com/

Reg and Maggie Green have established the Nicholas Green Foundation to increase awareness worldwide regarding the importance of organ donation.

Organ Donor Awareness Apparel
PO Box 18812
Tucson, AZ 85731
(520) 574-8358
(520) 574-8254 (fax)
DnRapparal@aol.com
http://www.i-netmall.com/shops/organdonor

Organ Donor Awareness Apparel is run by a family whose five-month-old daughter received a liver transplant. This is a good outlet for T-shirts, hats, and other items bearing slogans such as "Don't take your organs to heaven—heaven knows we need them here!"

The Partnership for Organ Donation
2 Oliver Street
Boston, MA 02109
(617) 482-5746
info@organ-donation.org
http://www.transweb.org/partnership/index.html

The Partnership for Organ Donation is an independent, non-profit organization dedicated to saving and improving lives by closing the gap between the number of organ transplants that are possible and the number of organ transplants that actually occur.

Second Wind Lung Transplant Association, Inc.
300 South Duncan Avenue, Suite 227
Clearwater, FL 33755-6457
(888) 222-2690 or (727) 442-0892
secondwind@netzero.net
http://www.2ndwind.org/

The Second Wind Lung Transplant Association, Inc. was established to improve the quality of life for lung transplant recipients, lung surgery candidates, people with related pulmonary concerns, and their families, by providing support, love, advocacy, education, information and guidance.

Transplant Awareness Inc.
PO Box 7634
Arlington, VA 22207
(888) 268-9232 or (703) 534-8587
(703) 534-7759 (fax)
tai01@aol.com
http://www.transplantawareness.org/

Transplant Awareness Inc. is a nonprofit corporation run and operated by volunteers who are all organ transplant recipients. Since TAI is run entirely by volunteers, one hundred percent of the profit from sales goes to increasing organ and tissue transplantation awareness. They sell bumper stickers, T-shirts, pins, keychains and other items bearing promotional slogans.

Transplant Recipients International Organization, Inc.
1000 16th Street, NW, Suite 602
Washington, DC 20036-5705
(800) TRIO-386 (874-6386) or (202) 293-0980
(202) 293 0973 (fax)
trio@primenet.com
http://www.trioweb.org/

The Transplant Recipients International Organization (TRIO) is an independent, not-for-profit, international organization committed to improving the quality of life of transplant candidates, recipients, their families and the families of organ and tissue donors.

TransWeb
The Northern Brewery Building
1327 Jones Drive, Suite 105
Ann Arbor, MI 48105
(734) 998-7314
(734) 998-6710 (fax)
transweb@umich.edu
http://www.transweb.org/

TransWeb is one of the premier Internet resources for transplant information. A charitable, non-profit organization, TransWeb is continually looking for volunteers.

The Wendy Marx Foundation
322 South Caroline SE
Suite 201
Washington, DC 20003
(202) 546-7270
WEMarx@aol.com
http://www.transweb.org/qa/qadon/donation_activities/marxfound.html

The Wendy Marx Foundation for Organ Donor Awareness is an all-volunteer, not-for-profit organization established to increase public awareness of the need for organ and tissue donation. Wendy Marx is a native of Rye Brook, NY, and a graduate of Duke University, and she now resides in San Francisco. In late 1989 at the age of 22, Ms. Marx suffered severe case of viral hepatitis B, which destroyed her liver. Her life was saved by a liver transplant. Foundation accomplishments include support of the US Transplant Games, funding of a medical fellowship for doctors who want to learn more about organ donation and transplantation, and development of the US Sports Council on Organ Donation, which includes athletes, sports journalists, and collegiate and professional coaches.

General

American Association of Tissue Banks
1350 Beverly Road
Suite 220-A
McLean, VA 22101
(703) 827-9582
(703) 356-2198 (fax)
aatb@aatb.org
http://www.aatb.org

Publishes ethical and technical standards and oversees the accreditation of tissue banks.

American Transplantation Association
47 W. Polk Street
PMB #100–140
Chicago, IL 60605
(800) 494-4527
ata@21stcentury.net

Division of Transplantation (US Health Resources and Services Administration)
5600 Fishers Lane
Room 7C-22
Parklawn Building
Rockville, MD 20857
(301) 443-7577
http://www.hrsa.dhhs.gov/osp/dot/

MedicAlert Foundation
2323 Colorado Avenue
Turlock, CA 95382
(800) ID-ALERT (432-5378)
http://www.medicalert.org/
Organization providing bracelets with emergency medical information and a contact for additional detailed information.

The Mickey Mantle Foundation
8080 N. Central Expressway
Suite 800
Dallas, TX 75206-1887
(800) 477-MICK (6425)
http://www.transweb.org/mantle.html

Working to eliminate the shortage of organs through awareness and education.

Minority Organ Tissue Transplant Education Program (MOTTEP)
2041 Georgia Avenue, NW
Suite 3100
Washington, DC 20060
(202) 865-4888
(800) 393-2839

NAACP Black Donor Education Program
4805 Mt. Hope Drive
Baltimore, MD 21215
(310) 358-8900

National Transplant Pregnancy Registry
c/o Dr. Vincent Armenti
Thomas Jefferson University
Department of Surgery—Transplant Program
1025 Walnut Street
Suite 605
Philadelphia, PA 19107
(215) 955-2840

United Network for Organ Sharing (UNOS)
PO Box 13770
1100 Boulders Parkway
Suite 500
Richmond, VA 23225-8770
(804) 330-8500
http://www.unos.org/

A private, non-profit corporation that administers organ procurement and distribution. UNOS manages the list of patients awaiting organ transplant and establishes policies for ensuring fair distribution. They maintain an extremely informative we site.

Specific organs and tissues

American Liver Foundation
75 Maiden Lane, Suite 603
New York, NY 10038
(800) GO LIVER (465-4837)
http://sadieo.ucsf.edu/alf/alffinal/homepagealf.html

Dedicated to preventing, treating and curing hepatitis and all liver diseases through research, education and support groups.

The Eye Bank Association of America
1001 Connecticut Ave NW Suite 601
Washington, DC 20036-5504
(202) 775-4999
(202) 429-6036 (fax)
http://www.restoresight.org/

Dedicated to restoring sight through the promotion and advancement of eye banking.

National Kidney Foundation
(800) 622-9010
transplant@kidney.org
http://www.kidney.org/recips/athletics/

Seeks to prevent kidney and urinary tract diseases, improve the health and well-being of individuals and families affected by these diseases, and increase the availability of all organs for transplantation. It also organizes the Transplant Games, a four-day athletic competition open to any recipient of a solid-organ or bone-marrow transplant.

Transplants in children

Children's Liver Alliance
(also known as the Biliary Atresia & Liver Transplant Network Inc.)
3835 Richmond Avenue, Box 190
Staten Island, NY 10312
(718) 987-6200
livers4kids@earthlink.net
http://www.livertx.org/

Provides information, support, and education to children, families, and the general public regarding liver disease.

Children's Liver Association for Support Services (CLASS)
26444 Emerald Dove Drive
Valencia, CA 91355
(877) 679-8256
(661) 255-0353
SupportSrv@aol.com
http://www.classkids.org/

An all-volunteer, nonprofit organization dedicated to serving the emotional, educational, and financial needs of families coping with childhood liver disease and transplantation.

Children's Organ Transplant Association
2701 COTA Drive
Bloomington, IN 47403
(800) 366-2682
http://www.cota.org/

Provides financial assistance for organ transplants, promotes organ donation awareness, and educates on all aspects of the organ donation process.

Financial

American Kidney Fund
6110 Executive Boulevard
Suite 1010
Rockville, Maryland 20852
(800) 638-8299 or (301) 881-3052
(301) 881-0898 (fax)
http://www.akfinc.org/

Provides financial assistance, support, and information to those suffering from kidney failure.

Barbara Anne DeBoer Foundation
2069 S. Busse Road
Mt. Prospect, IL 60056
(800) 895-8478
BADFDN@aol.com

National Foundation for Transplants
(formerly Organ Transplant Fund)
1102 Brookfield
Suite 200
Memphis, Tennessee 38119
(800) 489-3863 or (901) 684-1697
(901) 684-1128 (fax)
http://www.transplants.org

Offers a program of financial support services and patient advocacy for transplant candidates, recipients, and their families nationwide. Assists with fund-raising campaigns and grants.

National Transplant Assistance Fund
6 Bryn Mawr Avenue
PO Box 258
Bryn Mawr, PA, USA 19010
(800) 642-8399 or (610) 527-5056
(610) 527-5210 (fax)
http://www.transplantfund.org

Provides educational information, fund-raising expertise for patients raising money for transplants, and financial support to patients through medical assistance grants.

Physician organizations

American Society of Transplantation
(formerly American Society of Transplant Physicians)
6900 Grove Road
Thorofare, NJ 08086-9447
(856) 848-6205
http://www.a-s-t.org/index.htm

An organization of physicians dedicated to research, education, advocacy and patient care in transplantation science and medicine.

International Society for Heart and Lung Transplantation
14673 Midway Road
Suite 200
Addison, Texas 75001
(972) 490-9495
ishlt@ishlt.org
http://www.ishlt.org/

An organization of physicians dedicated to the advancement of science and treatment of heart and lung diseases.

Mail-order pharmacies

American Preferred Prescription, Inc. (APP)
50 Republic Road
Melville, NY 11747
(800) 227-1195
http://www.apprx.com/

Chronimed, Inc.
10900 Red Circle Drive
Minnetonka, MN 55343
(800) 888-5753
http://www.chronimed.com/

SangStat Medical Corporation
6300 Dumbarton Circle
Fremont, CA 94555
(888) 800-7264
http://www.sangstat.com/

Stadtlanders Pharmacy
600 Penn Center Boulevard
Pittsburgh, PA 15235
(800) 238-7828
http://www.stadtlander.com/

Financial assistance

Civilian Health and Medical Program of the Uniform Services (CHAMPUS)
(303) 361-1126

Medicare Hotline
(800) 638-6833

Social Security Administration
(800) 772-1213
http://www.ssa.gov/

Drug-company subsidies

Several pharmaceutical companies provide subsidies to patients in financial need. They are listed with their toll-free telephone numbers in the following table:

Drug	Manufacturer	Telephone Number
Bactrim	Roche	(800) 526-6367
Calan	Searle	(800) 542-2526
Cardizem	Marion Merrell Dow	(800) 552-3656

Drug	Manufacturer	Telephone Number
Dilantin	Parke-Davis	(800) 755-0120
Epogen, Neupogen	Amgen	(800) 272-9376
Imuran/zovirax	Burroughs Wellcome	(800) 722-9294
Sandimmune, Neoral	Novartis	(800) 447-6673
Vasotec, Prilosec Merck	Sharp & Dome	(800) 637-2579
Zantac	Glaxo	(800) 452-9677
Micronase	Upjohn	(616) 323-6004

State pharmaceutical-assistance programs

The following table provides toll-free numbers for organizational programs that provide pharmaceutical-assistance programs:

State	Organization	Telephone Number
	National Organization for State Kidney Programs	(800) 733-7345
CT	Connecticut Pharmaceutical Assistance Contract to the Elderly and the Disabled	(800) 423-5026
DE	The Nemours Health Clinic Program	New Castle: (302) 429-8050 Kent & Sussex: (800) 292-9538
IL	Pharmaceutical Assistance Programs	(800) 624-2459 or (217) 524-0435
ME	Elderly Low-Cost Drug Program	(800) 773-7894
MD	Pharmacy Assistance Program	(800) 492-1974
NJ	Pharmaceutical Assistance to the Aged and Disabled	(800) 792-9745
NY	EPIC Program	(800) 332-3742
PA	Pharmaceutical Assistance Contract for the Elderly	(800) 225-7223

Travel and lodging

AirLifeLine
6133 Freeport
Sacramento, CA 95822
(800) 446-1231

American Red Cross
(202) 728-6401

Angel Flight
American Medical Support Flight Team
3237 Donald Douglas Loop South
Santa Monica, CA 90405
(310) 398-6123

Mercy Medical Airlift (MMA)
(800) 296-1191

Mercy Medical Airlift's National Patient Air Transport Helpline (NPATH)
(800) 296-1217

Mission Air Transportation Network
(416) 222-6335

Mission Aviation Fellowship
(909) 794-1151

National Association of Hospital Hospitality Houses
(800) 542-9730

Ronald McDonald Houses
(312) 836-7100

Books and other publications

Books

Caplan, Arthur L., and Daniel H. Coehlo (editors). *The Ethics of Organ Transplantation: The Current Debate.* New York: Prometheus Books, 1998. This book contains a myriad of essays on the ethical, religious, and socio-cultural aspects of organ transplantation.

Chabot-Long, Lynn. *The Gift of Life: A Page From the Life of a Living Organ Donor.* Milwaukee: Je-Lynn Publications, 1996. Lynn Chabot-Long tells the story of her decision to donate a kidney to her brother.

Gutkind, Lee. *Many Sleepless Nights: The World of Organ Transplantation.* Pittsburgh: University of Pittsburgh Press, 1990. An excellent book focusing on a single transplant team and individual patients.

Keene, Nancy. *Working with Your Doctor: Getting the Healthcare You Deserve.* Sebastopol, California: O'Reilly & Associates, 1998. Another book in the Patient-Centered Guide series that may prove useful as you navigate your way through the medical system.

The Massachusetts General Hospital Organ Transplant Team and H. F. Pizer. *Organ Transplants: A Patient's Guide.* Cambridge: Harvard University Press, 1991. In addition to the book in your hands, here's another book that provides many of the everyday details of organ transplantation, especially as these details affect the day-to-day life of the transplant recipient. Although it is a bit out of date and covers less ground than the present book, I learned a great deal by reading it

McCartney, Scott. *Defying the Gods: Inside the New Frontiers of Organ Transplants.* New York: Macmillan Publishing Company, 1994. An excellent book focusing on a single transplant team and individual patients.

Oster, Nancy, and Lucy Thomas and Darol Joseff. *Making Informed Medical Decisions: Where to Look and How to Use What You Find.* Sebastopol, California: O'Reilly & Associates, 2000. An upcoming title in the Patient-Centered Guide series that may prove useful as you navigate your way through the medical system.

Shaffer, Marianne L., RN. *Bone Marrow Transplants: A Guide for Cancer Patients and Their Families.* Dallas: Taylor Publishing Company, 1994. For more on bone marrow transplants.

Starzl, Thomas E. *The Puzzle People: Memoirs of a Transplant Surgeon.* Pittsburgh: University of Pittsburgh Press, 1992. For more on the history of transplantation, see this fascinating personal account by Dr. Thomas E. Starzl, one of the field's foremost pioneers.

Youngner, Stuart J., and Renée C. Fox and Laurence J. O'Connell (editors). *Organ Transplantation: Meanings and Realities.* Madison: The University of Wisconsin Press, 1996. Another book containing essays on the ethical, religious, and sociocultural aspects of organ transplantation.

Zukerman, Eugenia, and Julie R. Inglefinger, MD. *Coping with Prednisone: It May Work Miracles, But How Do You Handle the Side Effects?* New York: St. Martin's Griffin, 1998. A fine book on prednisone, one of the main immunosuppressive medications.

Newsletters and journals

Blood & Marrow Transplant Newsletter
2900 Skokie Valley Road
Highland Park, IL 60035
(847) 433-3313
(888) 597-7674
http://www.bmtnews.org/

You'll find other good information on bone marrow transplants here (formerly *BMT Newsletter*).

Transplant Communications, Inc.
10 Rollins Road
Suite 106
Millbrae, CA 94030
(800) 689-4262
trannews@aol.com
http://www.trannews.com/

Published 24 times a year, *Transplant News* is the only independent newsletter covering the field. Jim Warren, its editor and publisher, also publishes the annual *International Transplant Directory.*

Transplant Video Journal
(973) 316-8800
transvidjr@aol.com

Free quarterly journal with informative updates of the latest transplant research and news. Phone or send email to subscribe.

Additional web sites

The Heart Failure Hotel
(tour a heart transplant unit)
http://www.homestead.com/alouso/

"HLA Matching, Antibodies, and You"
http://www.med.umich.edu/trans/public/hla/hla_&_you.html
A useful document from the University of Michigan Medical Center.

Jim Gleason's personal transplant account
http://transweb.org/people/recips/experien/gleason/

Lori Noyes's personal transplant account
http://www.geocities.com/HotSprings/2784/story1.html

The Lung Transplant Zone
http://members.aol.com/Mtrunn5402/siteintroduction.html

The Organ Transplant Ring
http://www.geocities.com/HotSprings/8374/start.html

Transplant Candidates' & Recipients' Own Web Pages
http://transweb.org/people/recips/pt_pages_index.html
A list of links to many transplant recipients informative and enlightening accounts of their experiences.

"Understanding Tissue Typing"
http://www.med.umich.edu/trans/public/ttbrochure/pg1.html
Another useful document from the University of Michigan Medical Center.

Internet support groups

Internet resources and addresses can change rapidly. In this section, we list only the most useful resources, and ones that we believe will be stable. Don't be dismayed if a particular address has changed. Go to a catalog of pages, such as *http://www.yahoo.com/*, or to a search engine such as *http://www.altavista.com/*, and look up the organization by name. You may also wish to take that opportunity to search for other resources on organ transplants.

Mailing lists

- TRNSPLNT. To subscribe, point your web browser to *http://www.concentric.net/~Holloway/* An alternate method is to send email to *listserv@wuvmd.wustl.edu*. In the body of the message, type the following single line (substituting your name): SUB TRNSPLNT Jane Doe.

- A list called txlongterm is intended for people who have been transplant recipients for extended periods. It concentrates on rehabilitation and unique physical issues for such people. To subscribe to txlongerm, go to *http://www.onelist.com/*.

- The DIALYSIS list is specifically for kidney patients. To subscribe, send mail to *listproc@mail.wustl.edu*. In the body of the message, type the following single line (substituting your name): subscribe DIALYSIS Jane Doe.

- If you are a spouse, family member, or caregiver of someone who is awaiting or is already a recipient of a lung transplant, you may wish to subscribe to the ASSIST mailing list. To do so, send email to *ASSIST-request@HOME.EASE. LSOFT.COM*.

  This message will be read by a real person, not an automated list processor. In your message, include your loved one's diagnosis, describe your relationship to that person (e.g., spouse, parent, sibling), and mention whether the person has already been transplanted or is waiting.

- The Second Wind National Lung Transplant Patient's Association maintains a discussion list for messages concerning lung diseases, lung transplants, problems, solutions, and "life in general." You'll find the subscription form at *http://www.2ndwind.org/join.htm*.

- If you are dealing with the long-term complications of years of diabetes, even after a kidney/pancreas transplant, you may wish to subscribe to the Kidney/Pancreas Support Group. To subscribe, send a blank email to: *kptx-subscribe@makelist.com*.

Chats

- For an up-to-date list of scheduled weekly chats organized by online service, see the TRNSPLNT FAQ available at *http://www.faqs.org/faqs/medicine/transplant-faq/part1/*.

- The Children's Liver Alliance currently hosts four separate chats rooms for adult family members, children (including siblings), medical professionals, and staff and volunteers. For more information, email *Livers4Kids@earthlink.net* or call (718) 987-6200. To find out more or to participate, go to the Alliance web site at *http://www.livertx.org*.

- If you have access to ICQ—special software that allows for real-time chats over the Internet—you may wish to register your ICQ number at the Organ Transplant Support Group Chat. Visiting this web page will allow you to contact about 100 transplant recipients (at last count) who have indicated a willingness to chat about their experiences. They can be found at: *http://www.jensoft-cs.com/icqlist.html*.

Notes

Chapter 1: *Considering a Transplant*

1. The source for all data in this section is the United Network for Organ Sharing (UNOS), the main national transplant organization in the United States. These figures refer only to people receiving transplants in the US. UNOS provides a wealth of data on transplants on its web site at *http://www.unos.org/*.
2. This is based in part on a document that was compiled by UNOS and which you can find at: *gopher://info.med.yale.edu:70/00/Disciplines/Disease/Transplant/religion.txt*.

Chapter 2: *The System*

1. Sheryl Gay Stolberg, "Fight over Organs Shifts to States from Washington," *New York Times*, 12 March 1999.

Chapter 9: *Living with a Transplant*

1. M. F. Mamzer-Bruneel et al., "Treatment and Prognosis of Post-Transplant Lymphoproliferative Disease," *Annals of Transplantation* 2 (1997): 42–48.

Chapter 11: *Family and Support*

1. Some of these items come from the "Checklist for Parenting Stressed Children" in: Nancy Keene and Rachel Prentice, *Your Child in the Hospital: A Practical Guide for Parents* (Sebastopol, California: O'Reilly & Associates, 1999): 79–80.

Chapter 13: *Living Donors*

1. Larry S. Goldman, "Liver Transplantation Using Living Donors: Preliminary Donor Psychiatric Outcomes," *Psychosomatics* 34 (1993): 235–40.
2. Lynn Chabot-Long, *The Gift of Life: A Page from the Life of a Living Organ Donor*, (Milwaukee: Je-Lynn Publications, 1996).
3. M. L. Barr et al., "Recipient and Donor Outcomes in Living Related and Unrelated Lobar Transplantation," *Transplantation Proceedings* 30 (1998): 2261-3.

Chapter 14: *Donors and Recipients*

1. Arthur L. Caplan, "Ethical and Policy Issues in the Procurement of Cadaver Organs for Transplantation," *The New England Journal of Medicine* 311 (1984): 981–83. Also in Caplan and Coelho, *The Ethics of Organ Transplants*, 142–46.

2. Aaron Spital, "Mandated Choice for Organ Donation: Time to Give It a Try," *Annals of Internal Medicine* 125 (1996): 66–69. Also in Caplan and Coelho, *The Ethics of Organ Transplants*, 147–53.

3. Ann C. Klassen and David K. Klassen, "Who Are the Donors in Organ Donation? The Family's Perspective in Mandated Choice," *Annals of Internal Medicine*, 125 (1996): 70–73. Also in Caplan and Coelho, *The Ethics of Organ Transplants*, 154–160.

4. Laurie G. Futterman, "Presumed Consent: The Solution to the Critical Donor Shortage?" *Alternative Therapies in Health and Medicine, American Journal of Critical Care* 4 (1995): 383–88. Also in Caplan and Coelho, *The Ethics of Organ Transplants*, 161–172.

5. R. M. Veatch and J. B. Pitt, "The Myth of Presumed Consent: Ethical Problems in New Organ Procurement Strategies," *Transplantation Proceedings* 27 (1995): 1888–92. Also in Caplan and Coelho, *The Ethics of Organ Transplants*, 173–182.

6. Thomas G. Peters, "Life or Death: The Issue of Payment in Cadaveric Organ Donation," *Journal of the American Medical Association* 265 (1991): 1302–5. Also in Caplan and Coelho, *The Ethics of Organ Transplants*, 196–204. Andrew H. Barnett, Roger D. Blair, and David L. Kaserman, "Improving Organ Donation: Compensation Versus Markets," *Inquiry* 2 (1993): 372–78. Also in Caplan and Coelho, *The Ethics of Organ Transplants*, 208–18.

7. Edmund D. Pellegrino, "Families' Self-Interest and the Cadaver's Organs: What Price Consent," *Journal of the American Medical Association*, 265 (1991): 1305–6. Also in Caplan and Coelho, *The Ethics of Organ Transplants*, 205–207. A. L. Caplan, C. T. Van Buren, and N. L. Tilney, "Financial Compensation for Cadaver Organ Donations: Good Idea or Anathema?" *Transplantation Proceedings* 25 (1993): 2740–42. Also in Caplan and Coelho, *The Ethics of Organ Transplants*, 219–23.

8. Rupert Jarvis, "Join the Club: A Modest Proposal to Increase Availability of Donor Organs," *Journal of Medical Ethics* 21 (1995): 199–204. Also in Caplan and Coelho, *The Ethics of Organ Transplants*, 183–192.

Chapter 15: *Financial Issues*

1. Lucette Lagnado, "Transplant Patients Ply Illicit Market for Drugs," *Wall Street Journal*, 21 June 1999.

Chapter 16: *Traveling for Treatment*

1. This chapter owes a great deal to a similar chapter in: Lorraine Johnston, *Non-Hodgkin's Lymphomas: Making Sense of Diagnosis, Treatment, and Options* (Sebastopol, California: O'Reilly and Associates, 1999).

Chapter 17: *The Future of Transplantation*

1. Lawrence K. Altman, "New Direction for Transplants Raises Hopes and Questions," *New York Times* (2 May 1999).

2. Michael J. Lysaght and Patrick Aebischer, "Encapsulated Cells as Therapy," *Scientific American* (April 1999): 76–82.

3. Robert Finn, "Reports Give Boost to Xenotransplantation as Researchers Wait for Federal Guidelines," *The Scientist* 10 (19 August 1996). This article is also available online at: *http://www.the-scientist.library.upenn.edu/yr1996/August/xeno_960819.html.*

4. An excellent series of reports on artificial hearts appeared on page A1 of the *Houston Chronicle* on October 12, 13, 14, and 15, 1997. Written largely by medical writer Ruth SoRelle, the series, called "Spare Hearts," is available online at *http://www.chron.com/content/chronicle/metropolitan/heart/.*

5. *Scientific American* published a series of informative articles on various aspects of tissue engineering in its April 1999 issue, which is available in most libraries.

Index

Internet sites, 4, 9–10, 192–197, 281–294
intestine transplants, 109–110, 229
intravenous pyelography (IVP), 221
Islamic teachings on transplants, 12
islet-cell transplants, 272–273

J

Jehovah's Witness teachings on transplants, 12
Judaism teachings on transplants, 12

K

Keefe, Emmet B.
    costs of transplantation, 246–247
    liver preservation and transportation, 89
    living related donors, 211
    multiple listings, 42
    organ distribution regulations, 40
    post-liver transplant activities, 92–93
    qualifying for liver transplants, 85–87
    recovery from liver donation surgery, 228–229
    splitting cadaveric livers, 88, 211
    support following transplant, 30
    surgeon experience and time on lists, 39
    use of anti-rejection drugs, 119
    waiting lists for liver transplants, 36–37
kidney and pancreas transplants, 94–106
    kidney transplants
        cost of, 33, 247–248 (chart)
        donor surgery, 220–226
        experimental alternative to, 274
        immediately after surgery, 103–104
        Medicare/Medicaid payment for, 33, 251–253
        number of, 97
        qualifying for, 97–99
        recipients, survival rates of, 3, 49, 211

recipients of, 94–97
recovery period following, 104–106
rejection, incidence of, 136
state subsidies for drugs, 263, 289–290 (chart)
surgical details of, 101–103
tests for candidates, 98–99
waiting list for, 37–38
pancreas and kidney-pancreas transplants
    cost of, 247–248 (chart)
    donor surgery, 229
    experimental alternative to, 273–274
    immediately after surgery, 103–104
    number of, 97
    qualifying for, 100–101
    recipients, survival rate of, 3
    recipients of, 94–97
    recovery period following, 104–106
    rejection, incidence of, 136
    surgical details of, 101–103
    waiting list for, 37–38
kidney list, 37–38
kidney-pancreas transplants. See kidney and pancreas transplants
kidney tomogram, 98
knee transplants, 272

L

laparoscopic nephrectomy, 223–226
learning about transplants, 7–10
left ventricular assist devices (LVADs), 277–278
Levin, Lisa G.
    avoiding infection, 151
    determining suitability of organs, 52–53
    patient responsibilities for self, 79, 148–149
    precautions with pets, 153
    travel by transplant recipients, 156–157
    travel to transplant centers, 53–54
ligament transplants, 113–114
limb transplants, 110–111

About the Author

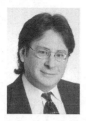

Robert Finn graduated from the University of Chicago with an AB in biological sciences, intending to pursue a career as a research neuroscientist. After several years of graduate studies at the University of California, Irvine, Department of Psychobiology, he realized he preferred writing to research. Robert left Irvine with an MS degree to pursue a career as a science writer. For a number of years, he worked full-time at the California Institute of Technology in Pasadena writing for Caltech's research magazine, and then for the news media, explaining scientific advances.

Since 1992, Robert has been a full-time freelance writer. His publication credits include articles for *Discover*, *Men's Fitness*, *OnHealth.com*, and *The Scientist* (where he was a contributing editor). Although he has written about many areas of science, he specializes in biomedicine and science policy. He has interviewed close to 1,000 scientists, physicians, and other experts during his career.

Organ Transplants: Making the Most of Your Gift of Life is Robert's second book. His first book, *Cancer Clinical Trials: Experimental Treatments and How They Can Help You*, is also published by O'Reilly.

Colophon

Patient-Centered Guides are about the experience of illness. They contain personal stories as well as a mixture of practical and medical information. The faces on the covers of our Guides reflect the human side of the information we offer.

The cover of *Organ Transplants: Making the Most of Your Gift of Life* was designed by Kathleen Wilson, Ellie Volckhausen, and Edie Freedman using Adobe Photoshop 5.0 and QuarkXPress 3.32 with Berkeley fonts from Bitstream. The cover photo is from Photodisc, and is used with that company's permission. The cover mechanical was prepared by Kathleen Wilson.

The interior layout for the book was designed by Alicia Cech, based on a design by Nancy Priest. The interior fonts are Berkeley and Franklin Gothic. The text was prepared by Alicia Cech and Mike Sierra using QuarkXPress 3.32 and FrameMaker 5.5. The text was copyedited by Lunaea Hougland and proofread by Sarah Jane Shangraw. Maureen Dempsey and Claire Cloutier provided quality assurance. The index was written by Kate Wilkinson. Interior composition was done by Sarah Jane Shangraw.

Robert Finn's photograph is from Hagop's Photography.

Patient-Centered Guides™

Questions Answered
Experiences Shared

We are committed to empowering individuals to evolve into informed consumers armed with the latest information and heartfelt support for their journey.

When your life is turned upside down, your need for information is great. You have to make critical medical decisions, often with what seems little to go on. Plus you have to break the news to family, quiet your own fears, cope with symptoms or treatment side effects, figure out how you're going to pay for things, and sometimes still get to work or get dinner on the table.

Patient-Centered Guides provide authoritative information for intelligent information seekers who want to become advocates of their own health. They cover the whole impact of illness on your life. In each book, there's a mix of:

- **Medical background for treatment decisions**
  We can give you information that can help you to intelligently work with your doctor to come to a decision. We start from the viewpoint that modern medicine has much to offer and also discuss complementary treatments. Where there are treatment controversies we present differing points of view.

- **Practical information**
  Once you've decided what to do about your illness, you still have to deal with treatments and changes to your life. We cover day-to-day practicalities, such as those you'd hear from a good nurse or a knowledgeable support group.

- **Emotional support**
  It's normal to have strong reactions to a condition that threatens your life or changes how you live. It's normal that the whole family is affected. We cover issues like the shock of diagnosis, living with uncertainty, and communicating with loved ones.

Each book also contains stories from both patients and doctors — medical "frequent flyers" who share, in their own words, the lessons and strategies they have learned when maneuvering through the often complicated maze of medical information that's available.

We provide information online, including updated listings of the resources that appear in this book. This is freely available for you to print out and copy to share with others, as long as you retain the copyright notice on the print-outs.

http://www.patientcenters.com

Other Books in the Series

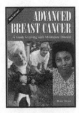

Advanced Breast Cancer
A Guide to Living with Metastatic Disease
By Musa Mayer
ISBN 1-56592-522-X, Paperback 6" x 9", 542 pages, $19.95

"An excellent book...if knowledge is power, this book will be good medicine."

—*David Spiegel, MD, Stanford University,*
Author, Living Beyond Limits

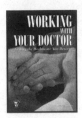

Working with Your Doctor
Getting the Healthcare You Deserve
By Nancy Keene
ISBN 1-56592-273-5, Paperback, 6" x 9", 382 pages, $15.95

"*Working with Your Doctor* fills a genuine need for patients and their family members caught up in this new and intimidating age of impersonal, economically-driven health care delivery."

—*James Dougherty, MD, Emeritus Professor of Surgery,*
Albany Medical College

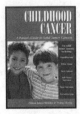

Childhood Cancer
A Parent's Guide to Solid Tumor Cancers
By Nancy Keene
ISBN 1-56592-531-9, Paperback, 6"x 9", 544 pages, $24.95

"I recommend [this book] most highly for those in need of high-level, helpful knowledge that will empower and help parents and caregivers to cope."

—*Mark Greenberg, MD, Professor of Pediatrics,*
University of Toronto

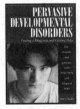

Pervasive Developmental Disorders
Finding a Diagnosis and Getting Help
By Mitzi Waltz
ISBN 1-56592-530-0, Paperback, 6" x 9", 592 pages, $24.95

"Mitzi Waltz's book provides clear, informative, and comprehensive information on every relevant aspect of PDD. Her in-depth discussion will help parents and professionals develop a clear understanding of the issues and, consequently, they will be able to make informed decisions about various interventions. A job well done!"

—*Dr. Stephen M. Edelson, Director,*
Center for the Study of Autism, Salem, Oregon

Patient-Centered Guides
Published by O'Reilly & Associates, Inc.
Our products are available at a bookstore near you.
For information: **800-998-9938** • **707-829-0515** • **info@oreilly.com**
101 Morris Street • Sebastopol • CA • 95472-9902

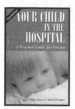

Your Child in the Hospital
A Practical Guide for Parents, Second Edition
By Nancy Keene and Rachel Prentice
ISBN 1-56592-573-4, Paperback, 5" x 8", 176 pages, $11.95

"When your child is ill or injured, the hospital setting can be overwhelming. Here is a terrific 'road map' to help keep families 'on track.'"

> —James B. Fahner, MD, Division Chief,
> Pediatric Hematology/Oncology, DeVos Children's Hospital,
> Grand Rapids, Michigan

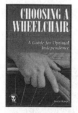

Choosing a Wheelchair
A Guide for Optimal Independence
By Gary Karp
ISBN 1-56592-411-8, Paperback, 5" x 8", 192 pages, $9.95

"I love the idea of putting knowledge often possessed only by professionals into the hands of new consumers. Gary Karp has done it. This book will empower people with disabilities to make informed equipment choices."

> —Barry Corbet, Editor, New Mobility Magazine

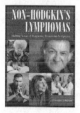

Non-Hodgkin's Lymphomas
Making Sense of Diagnosis, Treatment & Options
By Lorraine Johnston
ISBN 1-56592-444-4, Paperback, 6" x 9", 584 pages, $24.95

"When I gave this book to one of our patients, there was an instant, electric connection. A sense of enlightenment came over her while she absorbed the information. It was thrilling to see her so sparked with new energy and focus."

> —Susan Weisberg, LCSW, Clinical Social Worker,
> Stanford University Medical Center

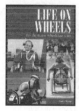

Life on Wheels
For the Active Wheelchair User
By Gary Karp
ISBN 1-56592-253-0, Paperback, 6" x 9", 576 pages, $24.95

"Gary Karp's Life On Wheels is a super book. If you use a wheelchair, you cannot do without it. It is THE wheelchair user reference book."

> —Hugh Gregory Gallagher, Author,
> FDR's Splendid Deception

Patient-Centered Guides
Published by O'Reilly & Associates, Inc.
Our products are available at a bookstore near you.
For information: **800-998-9938** • **707-829-0515** • **info@oreilly.com**
101 Morris Street • Sebastopol • CA • 95472-9902

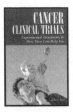

Cancer Clinical Trials
Experimental Treatments and How They Can Help You
By Robert Finn
ISBN 1-56592-566-1, Paperback, 5" x 8", 216 pages, $14.95

"I highly recommend this book as a first step in what will be for many a difficult, but crucially important, part of their struggle to beat their cancer."

—From the foreword by Robert Bazell, Chief Science
Correspondent for NBC News and Author,
Her-2: The Making of Herceptin, a Revolutionary
Treatment for Breast Cancer

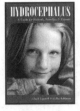

Hydrocephalus
A Guide for Patients, Families & Friends
By Chuck Toporek and Kellie Robinson
ISBN 1-56592-410-X, Paperback, 6" x 9", 384 pages, $19.95

"Toporek, a medical editor, and wife Robinson, a writer and hydrocephalus patient, fill a void of information on hydrocephalus (water on the brain) for the lay reader. Highly recommended for public and academic libraries."

—Library Journal

"In this book, the authors have provided a wonderful entry into the world of hydrocephalus to begin to remedy the neglect of this important condition. We are immensely grateful to them for their groundbreaking effort."

—Peter M. Black, MD, PhD, Franc D. Ingraham Professor of
Neurosurgery, Harvard Medical School,
Neurosurgeon-in-Chief, Brigham and Women's Hospital,
Children's Hospital, Boston, Massachusetts

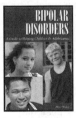

Bipolar Disorders
A Guide to Helping Children & Adolescents
By Mitzi Waltz
ISBN 1-56592-656-0, Paperback, 6" x 9", 450 pages, $24.95

"As bipolar disorders are becoming more commonly diagnosed in children and adolescents, a readable, informative guide for these youths and their families is certainly needed. This book certainly fits the bill. It covers all of the major topics that are of greatest importance to guide parents and families on the topic of pediatric bipolarity ..."

—Robert L. Findling, MD, Director, Division of Child and
Adolescent Psychiatry, Co-director, Stanley Clinical Research
Center, Case Western Reserve University/University
Hospitals of Cleveland

Patient-Centered Guides
Published by O'Reilly & Associates, Inc.
Our products are available at a bookstore near you.
For information: **800-998-9938** • **707-829-0515** • **info@oreilly.com**
101 Morris Street • Sebastopol • CA • 95472-9902

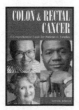

Colon & Rectal Cancer
A Comprehensive Guide for Patients & Families
By Lorraine Johnston
ISBN 1-56592-633-1, Paperback, 6" x 9", 530 pages, $24.95

"I sure wish [this book] had been available when I was first diagnosed.
I wouldn't change a thing: informative, down-to-earth, easily
understandable, and very touching."

—Pati Lanning, colon cancer survivor

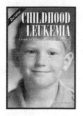

Childhood Leukemia
A Guide for Families, Friends, and Caregiver, 2nd Edition
By Nancy Keene
ISBN 1-56592-632-3, Paperback, 6" x 9", $24.95, 564 pages

"What's so compelling about Childhood Leukemia *is the amount of useful
medical information and practical advice it contains. Keene avoids jargon and
lays out what's needed to deal with the medical system."*

—The Washington Post

Patient-Centered Guides
Published by O'Reilly & Associates, Inc.
Our products are available at a bookstore near you.
For information: **800-998-9938** • **707-829-0515** • **info@oreilly.com**
101 Morris Street • Sebastopol • CA • 95472-9902